PACEMAKER

A Survival Guide For Patients

Dr. Bhratri Bhushan
MD, DM

To my father Dr. Bharat Bhushan

CONTENTS

PREFACE

In the intricate tapestry of human existence, the heart stands as both a resilient organ and a metaphorical compass guiding us through the rhythmic cadence of life. This book, a voyage into the realm of pacemakers for patients and caregivers, unfolds at the intersection of medical science and the human spirit.

In the opening chapters, we delve into the historical odyssey of pacemakers, tracing the evolution from the rudimentary external devices of the early 20th century to the cutting-edge, implantable technologies of today. As we unravel the threads of innovation, we encounter the pioneers and breakthroughs that have shaped the landscape of cardiac care.

A deeper exploration ensues, delving into the intricacies of the heart's anatomy and the common cardiac conditions that necessitate the intervention of these remarkable devices. The journey continues with an in-depth understanding of the role, types, and functioning of pacemakers, casting a spotlight on their pivotal role in restoring and regulating the heart's rhythm.

As we venture further, we navigate the procedural aspects of pacemaker implantation, from the meticulous preparation for the surgery to the nuanced recovery and post-implantation care. The narrative extends beyond the surgical theater, addressing the emotional and lifestyle considerations that accompany life with a pacemaker.

Lifestyle adjustments, dietary guidelines, and exercise considerations emerge as integral components of this holistic exploration, offering practical insights for individuals embarking on the post-implantation phase. We scrutinize the importance of regular follow-up, the advancements in remote monitoring technology, and the nuances of recognizing and addressing potential complications.

The narrative extends its embrace to the emotional impact of living with a pacemaker, acknowledging the resilience required to adapt to a new reality. Support systems, mental health considerations, and the communal strength derived from sharing experiences weave a fabric of understanding for both patients and caregivers.

In the later chapters, we venture into practical considerations, addressing the financial landscape, insurance coverage, and the significance of joining support networks. Emerging trends and innovations, including the integration of artificial intelligence, signal a future where pacemaker technology continues to evolve, promising even more personalized and efficient solutions.

Each chapter, a chapter in the chronicle of cardiac care, is a tapestry woven with insights, experiences, and a collective pursuit of well-being. As we embark on this journey, may this book serve as a compass, guiding patients and caregivers through the intricate terrain of pacemakers, and offering a beacon of hope, resilience, and empowerment.

Let the pages unfold, and may the rhythm of knowledge resonate with the beating hearts of those seeking understanding, support, and a roadmap to embrace life with a pacemaker.

INTRODUCTION

"I believe every human has a finite number of heartbeats. I don't intend to waste any of mine."
-Neil Armstrong

Historical background

The history of pacemakers is a testament to the continuous evolution of medical technology, marked by significant milestones and breakthroughs. The journey spans over a century, from the first inklings of understanding the heart's electrical system to the development of sophisticated, implantable devices that regulate cardiac rhythm. Here is a historical background of pacemakers:

1. Late 19th Century - Early 20th Century: Early Understanding of Cardiac Electrophysiology
   - The late 19th century witnessed crucial discoveries in cardiac electrophysiology. Pioneers like Augustus Waller and Willem Einthoven developed the electrocardiogram (ECG or EKG), allowing researchers to visualize the heart's electrical activity.

2. 1920s - 1930s: Beginning of External Pacing Experiments
   - Building on the understanding of

cardiac electrical signals, researchers began experimenting with external cardiac pacing. In 1928, Dr. Albert S. Hyman developed an external device that used a hand-cranked generator to deliver electrical impulses to the heart.

3. 1950s: The Invention of the First External Pacemaker
- In 1952, Dr. Paul Zoll introduced the first successful external pacemaker. This device, known as the "Zoll PM-65," was used to treat patients with Stokes-Adams attacks, a condition characterized by sudden loss of consciousness due to a heart block.

4. 1958: First Implantable Pacemaker
- Dr. Rune Elmqvist, a Swedish engineer, and Dr. Åke Senning, a cardiac surgeon, collaborated to develop the first implantable pacemaker. The device, known as the Elmqvist-Senning pacemaker, was implanted in a patient named Arne Larsson. This marked a significant shift from external to internal pacing.

5. 1960s: Transistor Technology and Miniaturization
- The advent of transistor technology in the 1960s facilitated the miniaturization of pacemakers. This development allowed for more practical and long-term implantable devices.

6. 1970s: Improvements in Battery Technology
- Advances in battery technology during the

1970s further enhanced the feasibility of long-term implantable pacemakers. Lithium batteries emerged, providing a more compact and efficient power source.

7. 1980s - 1990s: Dual-Chamber Pacemakers and Rate-Responsive Pacing

- The introduction of dual-chamber pacemakers in the 1980s allowed for more physiological pacing by coordinating the activity of both atria and ventricles. Rate-responsive pacing, which adjusts the heart rate based on the patient's physical activity, also became a standard feature.

8. Late 20th Century: Advances in Programming and Remote Monitoring

- The late 20th century saw improvements in pacemaker programming, allowing healthcare providers to tailor pacing parameters to individual patient needs. Additionally, remote monitoring technologies emerged, enabling healthcare professionals to monitor pacemaker function without the need for frequent in-person visits.

9. 21st Century: Leadless Pacemakers and Integration with Artificial Intelligence

- The 21st century brought about significant innovations, including leadless pacemakers that eliminate the need for traditional leads. Integration with artificial intelligence (AI) allows pacemakers to adapt to a patient's physiological needs more dynamically.

10. Ongoing Research and Future Directions

- Ongoing research focuses on regenerative medicine, gene therapy, and advanced energy-harvesting technologies. These endeavors aim to further enhance pacemaker technology, providing more sustainable and personalized solutions for patients with cardiac rhythm disorders.

The historical journey of pacemakers reflects a continual quest for improved cardiac care, driven by the convergence of medical knowledge, engineering innovations, and a commitment to enhancing the quality of life for individuals with heart rhythm disorders.

Importance of Understanding Pacemakers

In the realm of modern medicine, pacemakers stand as remarkable marvels of innovation, offering a lifeline to individuals grappling with cardiac rhythm disorders. As tiny electronic devices implanted in the chest, pacemakers play a pivotal role in regulating the heartbeat, ensuring a steady and healthy rhythm. The importance of understanding pacemakers cannot be overstated, as these devices not only serve as life-saving interventions but also significantly impact the quality of life for those who rely on them.

Life-Saving Intervention:

At the heart of the matter lies the life-saving potential of pacemakers. These devices are often prescribed for individuals suffering from bradycardia, a condition characterized by an abnormally slow heart rate. Understanding the intricate workings of pacemakers becomes a matter of life and death in these instances, as the device steps in to provide the necessary electrical impulses, ensuring that the heart beats at a rate sufficient to meet the body's demands.

Enhanced Quality of Life:
Beyond the immediate life-saving function, a profound understanding of pacemakers empowers individuals to actively engage in decisions regarding their cardiac health. Knowing the benefits and limitations of pacemakers allows patients to make informed choices about their treatment options, contributing to an improved quality of life. This informed decision-making process involves weighing the potential risks and benefits in consultation with healthcare professionals, fostering a sense of agency in the patient.

Preventing Complications:
A comprehensive understanding of pacemakers equips patients and caregivers with the knowledge to recognize and address potential complications. Proactive management of complications, such as infections or device malfunctions, becomes possible when individuals are well-informed. This

vigilance can prevent serious issues, safeguarding the patient's overall health and well-being.

Informed Decision-Making:
The decision to undergo pacemaker implantation is a significant one. Understanding the intricacies of the device allows patients to actively participate in this decision-making process. Armed with knowledge about the potential benefits and risks, individuals can make choices that align with their values and preferences, fostering a collaborative and patient-centered approach to healthcare.

Adherence to Lifestyle Guidelines:
Living with a pacemaker necessitates certain lifestyle adjustments. Whether it be considerations related to physical activity, diet, or other aspects of daily life, adherence to guidelines is crucial. Understanding the function and limitations of pacemakers enables patients to make informed choices, fostering a holistic approach to health and well-being.

Effective Communication with Healthcare Providers:
Patients who possess a thorough understanding of pacemakers can communicate more effectively with their healthcare providers. This communication extends beyond routine check-ups to include discussions about symptoms, concerns, and potential adjustments to the pacemaker settings. An open and informed

dialogue between patients and healthcare professionals is vital for optimal care and outcomes.

Reducing Anxiety and Fear:
A lack of understanding about pacemakers can lead to anxiety and fear. Clear and accessible information serves as a potent antidote to these emotions, providing reassurance and dispelling myths or misconceptions. Knowledgeable patients are better equipped to navigate their healthcare journey with confidence, reducing stress and enhancing overall well-being.

Promoting Patient Advocacy:
Understanding pacemakers transforms patients and caregivers into advocates for their own healthcare. Armed with knowledge, individuals can assert their needs and rights within the healthcare system. This advocacy extends beyond the individual to contribute to broader discussions about access to cardiac care and the importance of patient education.

Encouraging Compliance with Follow-up Care:
Regular follow-up care is paramount for individuals with pacemakers. Understanding the importance of follow-up appointments and remote monitoring encourages compliance. This diligence ensures that any issues, whether routine adjustments or potential concerns, are identified and addressed in a timely manner, contributing to

the long-term success of pacemaker therapy.

Building a Supportive Community:
An understanding of pacemakers fosters a sense of community among patients and caregivers who share similar experiences. This shared knowledge becomes the foundation for support networks where individuals can exchange information, offer advice, and provide emotional support. Building such a community is invaluable, as it creates a network of understanding and empathy among those navigating life with a pacemaker.

UNDERSTANDING THE HEART
AND CARDIAC CONDITIONS

"How frail the human heart must be—a mirrored pool of thought."
— Sylvia Plath

Anatomy of the Heart

The heart, with its rhythmic beats and tireless devotion to sustaining life, stands as the undisputed epicenter of the human circulatory system. This intricate organ, nestled within the chest, orchestrates a symphony of physiological processes that fuel the body's every movement. Embarking on a journey to understand the anatomy of the heart is to unravel the secrets of vitality, exploring the chambers, valves, and vessels that collaborate seamlessly to sustain the miracle of life.

The Heart's Position and Structure:
Positioned slightly to the left of the body's midline, the heart is a muscular organ enveloped in a protective sac known as the pericardium. Its structure is an architectural marvel, consisting of four chambers - two atria and two ventricles. The right atrium receives deoxygenated blood from the body, while the left atrium welcomes oxygenated

blood from the lungs. This demarcation sets the stage for a rhythmic dance that propels blood through a complex network of vessels.

Chambers and Valves:
The heart's chambers, each with a distinct role, are separated by valves that act as gatekeepers, ensuring the unidirectional flow of blood. The atrioventricular (AV) valves - the tricuspid valve on the right side and the bicuspid or mitral valve on the left - regulate the passage of blood between the atria and ventricles. Meanwhile, the pulmonary and aortic valves guard the exit points from the heart, directing blood towards the lungs and the rest of the body, respectively.

Blood Flow:
Understanding the anatomy of the heart is synonymous with comprehending the orchestrated ballet of blood flow. Deoxygenated blood returning from the body enters the right atrium through the superior and inferior vena cava. It then traverses the tricuspid valve into the right ventricle, which contracts to propel the blood through the pulmonary valve into the pulmonary artery, destined for oxygenation in the lungs. The freshly oxygenated blood returns to the left atrium via the pulmonary veins, flows through the mitral valve into the left ventricle, and is ejected into the aorta to circulate throughout the body.

The Heart's Musculature:

At the heart of the heart's function lies its muscular composition. The myocardium, a specialized muscle tissue, is responsible for the organ's powerful contractions. These contractions, driven by electrical impulses, create the force necessary to pump blood efficiently. The myocardium is a testament to the heart's endurance, tirelessly contracting and relaxing throughout a lifetime.

Coronary Circulation:
Even the heart, the emblem of vitality, requires its own supply of oxygen and nutrients. Coronary arteries, arising from the aorta, intricately weave across the heart's surface, providing the myocardium with the nourishment it needs. Any compromise in this coronary circulation can lead to serious consequences, highlighting the critical role of these vessels in maintaining the heart's health.

Heart's Electrical System:
The heart's rhythmic beats are orchestrated by its internal electrical system. The sinoatrial (SA) node, often referred to as the heart's natural pacemaker, initiates electrical impulses that travel through the atria, prompting them to contract. The impulses then pass through the atrioventricular (AV) node before traversing the bundle of His and Purkinje fibers, inducing ventricular contraction. This synchronized electrical symphony ensures the rhythmic

coordination of the heart's chambers.

The Heart as a Vital Organ:
Beyond its physiological intricacies, the heart symbolizes vitality, love, and resilience. The profound understanding of its anatomy is not only a pursuit of scientific knowledge but a journey into the very essence of human existence. As a vital organ, the heart sustains life, and as a symbol, it encapsulates the emotions and experiences that make us uniquely human.

Common Cardiac Conditions Requiring Pacemakers

The human heart, a marvel of biological engineering, orchestrates the symphony of life, maintaining a rhythmic beat that propels blood throughout the body. However, this vital organ is not immune to malfunctions, and certain cardiac conditions may disrupt its natural rhythm. In these instances, pacemakers emerge as crucial medical interventions, providing the necessary electrical support to restore and regulate the heartbeat. This essay delves into the intricacies of common cardiac conditions that often necessitate the use of pacemakers, shedding light on the significance of these devices in managing and preserving cardiovascular health.

Bradycardia:

One of the primary cardiac conditions that often leads to pacemaker implantation is bradycardia, characterized by an abnormally slow heart rate. Bradycardia can result from aging, heart damage, or certain medical conditions. When the heart's natural pacemaker, the sinoatrial (SA) node, fails to generate electrical impulses at the required rate, bradycardia can ensue. Pacemakers become indispensable in these cases, as they deliver timely electrical signals to stimulate the heart, ensuring a regular and sufficient heartbeat.

Heart Block:
Heart block is another cardiac condition that may necessitate pacemaker intervention. This condition arises when the electrical signals generated by the SA node face obstacles or delays as they traverse the heart's conduction system. Classified into first, second, and third degrees, heart block can significantly disrupt the synchronization between the atria and ventricles. Pacemakers address this issue by providing artificial signals, ensuring a coordinated and efficient heartbeat despite the electrical disturbances.

Sick Sinus Syndrome:
Sick Sinus Syndrome (SSS) is a collective term for a group of rhythm disorders originating from the sinus node. This condition manifests as alternating episodes of bradycardia and tachycardia, leading to an unpredictable

and irregular heartbeat. Pacemakers are often prescribed for individuals with SSS to maintain a stable heart rate and prevent potentially dangerous pauses or accelerations in the heartbeat.

Atrial Fibrillation and Atrial Flutter:
Atrial fibrillation (AFib) and atrial flutter are conditions characterized by irregular and often rapid heartbeats originating from the atria. While pacemakers themselves may not be the primary treatment for these arrhythmias, they are sometimes used in conjunction with other devices, such as implantable cardioverter-defibrillators (ICDs), to manage the overall rhythm of the heart.

Post-Cardiac Surgery Arrhythmias:
In the aftermath of cardiac surgeries, some patients may experience temporary arrhythmias due to the surgical manipulation of the heart's conduction system. Pacemakers are employed as a temporary measure to stabilize the heartbeat during the postoperative period until normal rhythm is restored.

Whether addressing bradycardia, heart block, sick sinus syndrome, or post-cardiac surgery arrhythmias, pacemakers serve as invaluable tools in the hands of healthcare professionals, providing patients with a lifeline to normal cardiac function.

Role of the Pacemaker
in Cardiac Health

This section explores the profound and pivotal role of the pacemaker in cardiac health, delving into how this small electronic device becomes a lifeline for individuals grappling with rhythm disturbances.

Restoring Rhythmic Order:
At the heart of the matter lies the primary function of the pacemaker — to restore and maintain the heart's natural rhythm. When the heart's intrinsic pacemaker, the sinoatrial (SA) node, falters, leading to bradycardia or other arrhythmias, the pacemaker steps in as a surrogate conductor. By delivering precisely timed electrical impulses, the pacemaker ensures that the heart contracts at a regular rate, allowing for efficient blood circulation and preventing complications associated with irregular heartbeats.

Addressing Bradycardia:
Bradycardia, characterized by a slow heart rate, is a common cardiac condition that underscores the essential role of pacemakers. Whether due to aging, heart damage, or certain medical conditions, bradycardia can compromise blood flow to vital organs. The pacemaker becomes a guardian in these instances, providing the

necessary stimuli to prompt the heart to beat at a rate that sustains life.

Managing Heart Block:
Heart block, a condition where electrical signals face delays or interruptions as they traverse the heart's conduction system, poses a significant threat to cardiac health. Pacemakers effectively manage heart block by delivering artificial signals that bridge the communication gaps, ensuring that the atria and ventricles coordinate their contractions and maintain the essential synchrony of the heartbeat.

Dynamic Adaptability in Sick Sinus Syndrome:
Sick Sinus Syndrome (SSS), a complex disorder involving the sinus node's inability to regulate the heart's rhythm, requires a dynamic and adaptive intervention. Pacemakers offer a tailored solution, adjusting their pacing based on the heart's needs. This adaptability is particularly crucial in SSS, where the heart experiences unpredictable shifts between bradycardia and tachycardia.

Ensuring Stability Post-Cardiac Surgery:
In the aftermath of cardiac surgeries, temporary arrhythmias may arise, disrupting the heart's natural rhythm. Pacemakers play a pivotal role in maintaining stability during this critical period, providing a steady beat until the heart's conduction system recovers from the surgical interventions.

Beyond Rhythm: Addressing Complex Arrhythmias:

While pacemakers primarily address bradycardia and certain rhythm disturbances, their role extends beyond restoring a regular heartbeat. In some cases, pacemakers work in conjunction with other devices, such as implantable cardioverter-defibrillators (ICDs), to manage complex arrhythmias like atrial fibrillation (AFib) or atrial flutter. This collaborative approach ensures comprehensive cardiac care for individuals facing multifaceted rhythm disorders.

Patient-Centered Care and Quality of Life:

Beyond the physiological impact, the pacemaker plays a crucial role in enhancing the quality of life for individuals with cardiac conditions. By restoring and maintaining a stable heart rate, pacemakers allow patients to engage in regular activities, exercise, and lead fulfilling lives. This patient-centered approach contributes to not only physical well-being but also mental and emotional health.

WHAT IS A PACEMAKER?

"Any sufficiently advanced technology is indistinguishable from magic."
-Arthur C. Clarke

Definition and Purpose

The heart, a marvel of biological engineering, serves as the life-sustaining rhythm that orchestrates the symphony of the human body. However, when the heart's natural pacemaker falters, an electronic marvel known as the pacemaker steps in as a guardian of life's pulsating melody.

Defining the Pacemaker:
A pacemaker is a small, implantable medical device designed to regulate and control the rhythm of the heart. It acts as an artificial pacemaker, generating electrical impulses to stimulate the heart to contract and pump blood effectively. Often implanted just beneath the skin in the chest, with leads extending into the heart chambers, the pacemaker becomes a silent conductor, ensuring that the heart maintains a steady and synchronized beat.

Purpose of the Pacemaker:

The primary purpose of a pacemaker is to address disturbances in the heart's natural electrical conduction system, which may result in irregular heartbeats or bradycardia (a slow heart rate). This critical intervention becomes necessary when the heart's intrinsic pacemaker, the sinoatrial (SA) node, fails to generate electrical impulses at the required rate or when electrical signals encounter obstacles or delays as they traverse the heart's conduction system.

Restoring and Maintaining Rhythm:
At its core, the pacemaker is a rhythm regulator, stepping in to restore and maintain the heart's natural beat. When the heart experiences bradycardia, characterized by a heart rate too slow to sustain life, the pacemaker emits electrical impulses, effectively instructing the heart to contract and pump blood. By ensuring a regular heartbeat, the pacemaker prevents complications associated with irregular rhythms and contributes to the overall stability of the cardiovascular system.

Adaptable Responses in Dynamic Conditions:
Pacemakers are designed with adaptability in mind, responding dynamically to the changing needs of the heart. This flexibility is particularly crucial in conditions such as Sick Sinus Syndrome (SSS), where the heart rhythm alternates between bradycardia and tachycardia. Pacemakers adjust their pacing based on the heart's requirements,

providing a customized solution to the complexities of cardiac rhythm disorders.

Addressing Heart Block and Conduction Disorders: Another vital purpose of the pacemaker is to address heart block and other conduction disorders. When electrical signals encounter obstacles or delays in their journey through the heart, the pacemaker serves as a bridge, delivering artificial signals to ensure that the atria and ventricles contract in a synchronized and coordinated manner. This intervention is crucial in preventing complications arising from the disruption of the heart's natural conduction system.

Enhancing Quality of Life:
Beyond its physiological functions, the pacemaker significantly enhances the quality of life for individuals with cardiac rhythm disorders. By restoring a regular heartbeat, the pacemaker allows patients to engage in regular activities, exercise, and lead fulfilling lives. This patient-centered approach contributes not only to physical well-being but also to mental and emotional health, fostering a sense of normalcy and empowerment.

Types of Pacemakers

The diversity of cardiac conditions and patient

needs has led to the development of various types of pacemakers, each tailored to address specific challenges. Following is an exploration of the types of pacemakers, unraveling the nuances of their designs, functionalities, and applications.

Single-Chamber Pacemakers:
Single-chamber pacemakers, as the name suggests, are designed to stimulate either the atria or the ventricles of the heart. In cases where the atria are the primary concern, an atrial pacemaker is implanted to regulate the heart's upper chambers. Similarly, a ventricular pacemaker is focused on stimulating the heart's lower chambers. Single-chamber pacemakers are often employed when only one part of the heart requires pacing, and they are chosen based on the specific needs of the individual patient.

Dual-Chamber Pacemakers:
In scenarios where both the atria and ventricles require pacing assistance, dual-chamber pacemakers emerge as versatile solutions. These pacemakers coordinate the pacing of both the upper and lower chambers, facilitating a more synchronized and natural heartbeat. Dual-chamber pacemakers mimic the heart's intrinsic conduction system more closely, enhancing the efficiency of blood flow and optimizing cardiac function.

Biventricular (CRT) Pacemakers:

Congestive heart failure often results in a lack of coordination between the heart's chambers, leading to compromised pump function. Biventricular pacemakers, also known as Cardiac Resynchronization Therapy (CRT) pacemakers, address this issue by stimulating both ventricles simultaneously. By synchronizing the contractions of the left and right ventricles, CRT pacemakers improve the heart's pumping efficiency, providing significant benefits for individuals with heart failure.

Rate-Responsive Pacemakers:
Rate-responsive pacemakers are equipped with sensors that monitor the body's physical activity and adjust the heart rate accordingly. These sensors, often responsive to factors such as body movement or respiration rate, enable the pacemaker to adapt to the individual's changing needs. Rate-responsive pacemakers are particularly beneficial for patients who lead active lifestyles, ensuring that the heart rate adjusts appropriately during exercise or periods of increased activity.

Leadless Pacemakers:
Traditional pacemakers involve the implantation of leads (thin wires) to deliver electrical impulses to the heart. Leadless pacemakers, a more recent innovation, eliminate the need for leads altogether. Instead, a small, self-contained device is directly implanted into the heart. Leadless

pacemakers reduce the risk of complications associated with traditional lead placement, offering a more streamlined and minimally invasive alternative.

MRI-Compatible Pacemakers:
Many individuals with pacemakers face limitations when it comes to undergoing magnetic resonance imaging (MRI) scans due to potential interference with the device. MRI-compatible pacemakers address this issue by incorporating designs that allow for safe MRI procedures. These devices provide individuals with pacemakers greater access to diagnostic imaging without compromising the functionality of the pacemaker.

How Pacemakers Work

For those whose hearts falter in maintaining this rhythm, pacemakers emerge as electronic maestros, orchestrating the heart's symphony. This chapter embarks on a detailed exploration of the mechanisms underlying how pacemakers work.

The Heart's Intrinsic Rhythm:
Before understanding the role of pacemakers, it is crucial to appreciate the heart's natural rhythm. The sinoatrial (SA) node, nestled in the right atrium, serves as the heart's intrinsic pacemaker.

This tiny cluster of cells generates electrical impulses that initiate each heartbeat. These impulses travel through the heart's conduction system, coordinating the sequential contractions of the atria and ventricles, ultimately propelling blood throughout the body.

Pacemakers as Artificial Conductors:
When the heart's natural pacemaker falters due to conditions like bradycardia or heart block, pacemakers step in as artificial conductors. These small devices, typically implanted beneath the skin in the chest, consist of a generator and leads. The generator houses the electronic circuitry and power source, while the leads extend into the heart, delivering precisely timed electrical impulses.

Generation of Electrical Impulses:
The pacemaker's generator contains a battery and electronic circuitry that work in unison to generate electrical impulses. These impulses mimic the natural signals produced by the SA node. The pacemaker is programmed to ensure that these signals are delivered at the appropriate rate to regulate the heartbeat. The ability to adjust pacing parameters makes pacemakers versatile instruments that can be tailored to the specific needs of individual patients.

Lead Placement and Sensing:
Leads, thin insulated wires, play a pivotal role

in pacemaker functionality. They are strategically placed in the heart to deliver electrical impulses to the atria, ventricles, or both, depending on the type of pacemaker. Additionally, the leads are equipped with sensors that can detect the heart's intrinsic electrical activity. This sensing capability allows the pacemaker to adapt its pacing to the heart's natural signals, creating a more physiologically responsive rhythm.

Mode Switching and Rate Responsiveness:
Modern pacemakers often incorporate advanced features such as mode switching and rate responsiveness. Mode switching allows the pacemaker to detect and respond to changes in the heart's electrical activity, switching between pacing modes as needed. Rate-responsive pacemakers utilize sensors to monitor factors like physical activity or respiration rate, adjusting the heart rate accordingly. This adaptive mechanism ensures that the heart responds dynamically to the body's changing needs.

Communication and Programming:
Pacemakers are equipped with sophisticated communication capabilities that allow healthcare professionals to monitor and adjust their settings remotely. This is particularly valuable for follow-up care, as it enables healthcare providers to assess pacemaker function, detect any issues, and make necessary adjustments without requiring physical intervention. Pacemakers are programmed during

implantation and can be reprogrammed as needed during follow-up appointments.

Battery Life and Replacement:
The longevity of a pacemaker is determined by its battery life, which can vary depending on factors such as pacing requirements and energy consumption. When the battery approaches the end of its life, the entire pacemaker is replaced through a relatively straightforward procedure. Regular check-ups and remote monitoring help healthcare providers assess battery status and plan for timely replacements.

INDICATIONS FOR PACEMAKER IMPLANTATION

"Technology is a gift of God. After the gift of life it is perhaps the greatest of God's gifts. It is the mother of civilizations, of arts and of sciences."
-Freeman Dyson

Medical Conditions Requiring Pacemakers

When the symphony of heartbeats encounters disruptions, medical conditions requiring pacemakers become critical focal points in cardiac care. Now we will discuss various medical conditions that necessitate the intervention of pacemakers, shedding light on the crucial role these devices play in restoring and maintaining the heartbeat.

Bradycardia:
Bradycardia, characterized by an abnormally slow heart rate, is a primary medical condition that often necessitates the use of pacemakers. As individuals age or encounter heart-related issues, the natural pacemaker, the sinoatrial (SA) node, may fail to generate electrical impulses at an adequate rate. Pacemakers become indispensable

in these cases, delivering timely electrical signals to stimulate the heart and ensure a regular and sufficient heartbeat.

Heart Block:
Heart block is a condition characterized by the interruption or delay of electrical signals as they traverse the heart's conduction system. This disruption in the coordination between the atria and ventricles can lead to a slow or irregular heartbeat. Pacemakers are employed to bridge the gaps in electrical signaling, ensuring that the heart chambers contract in a synchronized manner and maintain the essential harmony required for effective blood circulation.

Sick Sinus Syndrome (SSS):
Sick Sinus Syndrome is a collective term encompassing various rhythm disorders originating from the sinus node. This condition manifests as an alternating pattern of bradycardia and tachycardia, leading to an unpredictable and irregular heartbeat. Pacemakers play a pivotal role in managing SSS, providing artificial signals to regulate the heart rate and ensure a stable rhythm.

Atrial Fibrillation (AFib) and Atrial Flutter:
Atrial fibrillation and atrial flutter are arrhythmias characterized by irregular and often rapid heartbeats originating from the atria. While pacemakers themselves may not be the primary treatment for these conditions,

they are sometimes used in conjunction with other devices, such as implantable cardioverter-defibrillators (ICDs), to manage the overall rhythm of the heart. In some cases, pacemakers may be employed to address slow heart rates that can accompany these arrhythmias.

Post-Cardiac Surgery Arrhythmias:
In the aftermath of cardiac surgeries, some patients may experience temporary arrhythmias due to the surgical manipulation of the heart's conduction system. Pacemakers are utilized as a temporary measure to stabilize the heartbeat during the postoperative period until normal rhythm is restored. This ensures that the heart remains in a controlled and stable state as it recovers from the surgical intervention.

Certain Types of Heart Failure:
In specific cases of heart failure where there is a lack of coordination between the heart's chambers, leading to inefficient pumping, pacemakers known as biventricular pacemakers or Cardiac Resynchronization Therapy (CRT) pacemakers may be employed. These devices stimulate both ventricles simultaneously, improving the coordination of contractions and enhancing the heart's pumping efficiency.

Symptoms that May Indicate the Need for a Pacemaker

The following text embarks on a comprehensive exploration of symptoms that may indicate the need for a pacemaker, unraveling the subtle cues that prompt healthcare professionals to intervene and restore the heart's rhythmic harmony.

Bradycardia:
A primary indication for a pacemaker arises when the heart's rhythm slows down abnormally, a condition known as bradycardia. Symptoms associated with bradycardia often include fatigue, weakness, dizziness, and fainting spells. These manifestations occur as a consequence of insufficient blood flow to the organs and brain, highlighting the need for a pacemaker to restore a regular and adequate heartbeat.

Syncopal Episodes:
One of the more pronounced symptoms that may necessitate a pacemaker is syncope, or fainting. Syncopal episodes occur when the brain is temporarily deprived of oxygen due to a slow or irregular heart rate. Individuals experiencing recurrent fainting spells may undergo diagnostic assessments to determine if a pacemaker is required to address the underlying bradycardia or other rhythm disturbances.

Dyspnea:
A compromised heart rhythm can impact the efficient pumping of blood, leading to symptoms such as dyspnea or shortness of breath. When the

heart fails to maintain an adequate pace, the body struggles to meet the oxygen demands, resulting in breathlessness. Pacemakers play a crucial role in rectifying the rhythm, alleviating dyspnea, and improving overall cardiovascular function.

Fatigue and Weakness:
Bradycardia and other rhythm disturbances can contribute to persistent fatigue and weakness. The heart's inability to pump blood efficiently means that vital organs and muscles receive reduced oxygen and nutrients. These symptoms, when unexplained by other factors, may prompt healthcare professionals to investigate the possibility of pacemaker intervention.

Chest Discomfort:
Individuals experiencing disturbances in their heart rhythm may report chest discomfort or pain. While this symptom is not exclusive to rhythm disorders, its presence, especially when accompanied by other indicators, warrants careful evaluation. A thorough examination, including diagnostic tests, may reveal whether a pacemaker is necessary to restore the heart's natural harmony.

Palpitations:
Palpitations, a heightened awareness of one's heartbeat, can signal irregularities in heart rhythm. While palpitations can have various causes, persistent and unexplained occurrences

may prompt further investigation. Pacemakers are instrumental in addressing irregular heartbeats and restoring the steady rhythm necessary for optimal cardiovascular function.

Dizziness and Lightheadedness:

Dizziness and lightheadedness are common symptoms associated with disrupted heart rhythm. When the heart fails to pump blood efficiently, especially during position changes or physical exertion, inadequate blood flow to the brain can lead to these symptoms. A pacemaker becomes a therapeutic intervention to stabilize heart rate and alleviate these distressing sensations.

PACEMAKER IMPLANTATION PROCEDURE

"Let's have days and days of brilliant clarity, etched and limpid, cool and surgical."
-Richard Burton

Preparing for the Procedure

Introduction:
Pacemaker implantation, a medical procedure that involves the placement of a small electronic device to regulate and coordinate the heart's rhythm, is a transformative intervention for individuals facing cardiac rhythm disorders. This text provides an exploration of the preparatory steps and considerations involved in getting ready for the procedure of pacemaker implantation, ensuring a harmonious experience for both patients and healthcare providers.

Patient Evaluation and Consultation:
The journey towards pacemaker implantation begins with a thorough evaluation and consultation between the patient and the healthcare team. Cardiologists, electrophysiologists, and other specialists collaborate to assess the patient's medical

history, conduct a comprehensive physical examination, and perform diagnostic tests such as electrocardiograms (ECGs) and echocardiograms. This process helps determine the underlying rhythm disorder and whether a pacemaker is the appropriate course of action.

Informed Consent:
Once the decision for pacemaker implantation is made, the healthcare team engages in a crucial step—obtaining informed consent. Patients are provided with detailed information about the procedure, including its purpose, potential risks, benefits, and alternative treatment options. This ensures that individuals have a clear understanding of the intervention and actively participate in the decision-making process.

Pre-procedural Assessments:
In the days leading up to pacemaker implantation, patients undergo a series of pre-procedural assessments to ensure optimal conditions for the intervention. Blood tests, chest X-rays, and electrocardiograms may be performed to assess the patient's overall health, identify any potential contraindications, and assist in tailoring the procedure to the individual's specific needs.

Medication Management:
Patients may be advised to make adjustments to their medication regimen in the days preceding pacemaker implantation. Certain medications,

such as anticoagulants or antiplatelet agents, may need to be temporarily discontinued or adjusted to minimize the risk of bleeding during the procedure. Clear communication between the patient and healthcare team ensures a seamless transition in medication management.

Fasting and Lifestyle Considerations:
To create an optimal setting for the procedure, patients are typically instructed to fast for a specific period before the scheduled implantation. This helps minimize the risk of complications, especially those related to anesthesia. Additionally, lifestyle considerations, such as refraining from smoking and abstaining from alcohol, are often emphasized to promote overall well-being and support a successful pacemaker implantation.

Anesthesia and Sedation Options:
Pacemaker implantation is commonly performed under local anesthesia, with the option for conscious sedation. Local anesthesia numbs the implantation site, ensuring that patients do not experience pain during the procedure. Conscious sedation, administered through intravenous medications, induces a state of relaxation and drowsiness, allowing patients to remain conscious while alleviating anxiety and discomfort.

Placement and Positioning:
The actual procedure of pacemaker implantation

involves creating a small incision, usually in the upper chest, through which the pacemaker leads are threaded into the heart. The pacemaker generator, housing the electronic components and battery, is then secured beneath the skin. The precise placement of leads and generator, along with the choice of chambers to be paced, is determined based on the patient's specific rhythm disorder.

Post-procedural Care:
Following pacemaker implantation, patients are monitored closely in a recovery area. The healthcare team assesses vital signs, checks the implantation site for any signs of complications, and ensures that patients are comfortable. Once deemed stable, patients are provided with post-procedural care instructions, including guidelines for resuming activities, caring for the implantation site, and scheduling follow-up appointments.

The Surgical Process

This chapter provides a comprehensive exploration of the surgical process of pacemaker implantation, delving into the meticulous steps involved in orchestrating this life-enhancing intervention.

Preoperative Preparation:

Before the surgical process commences, patients undergo a series of preoperative preparations to ensure a smooth and successful implantation. This includes thorough patient evaluation, informed consent, and pre-procedural assessments to assess overall health and identify any potential contraindications. The collaborative efforts of the healthcare team aim to create an individualized plan tailored to the patient's specific needs.

Anesthesia Administration:
Pacemaker implantation is typically performed under local anesthesia, with the option for conscious sedation. Local anesthesia is administered to numb the surgical site, ensuring that patients do not experience pain during the procedure. Conscious sedation, delivered through intravenous medications, induces a state of relaxation and drowsiness, providing comfort and minimizing anxiety without the need for general anesthesia.

Surgical Incision:
The surgical process commences with the creation of a small incision, usually in the upper chest region. This incision serves as the gateway for accessing the subclavian vein, through which the pacemaker leads will be threaded into the heart. The size and location of the incision are carefully chosen to minimize scarring and promote optimal healing.

Lead Placement:
Once the incision is made, the next crucial step involves threading the pacemaker leads into the heart. The leads are thin, insulated wires equipped with electrodes that will deliver electrical impulses to stimulate the heart. The placement of leads is guided by fluoroscopy, a real-time X-ray imaging technique that allows the healthcare team to navigate the conduction pathways and position the leads accurately.

Pacemaker Generator Implantation:
With the leads in place, the pacemaker generator, containing the electronic circuitry and battery, is implanted beneath the skin. The generator is typically secured in a pocket created just beneath the incision site. This housing protects the delicate components of the pacemaker and facilitates easy access for future adjustments or replacements.

Testing and Verification:
After lead placement and generator implantation, the surgical team conducts thorough testing to ensure the pacemaker functions as intended. This involves verifying the electrical signals delivered by the leads, assessing the heart's response to pacing, and confirming the proper functioning of the pacemaker's programming. Real-time testing is crucial for making immediate adjustments and ensuring the device's efficacy.

Suture and Closure:

Once the testing phase is successfully completed, the surgical team proceeds to suture the incision site, concluding the implantation process. Sutures or adhesive strips may be used to close the incision, and a sterile dressing is applied to protect the site as it heals. The meticulous closure of the incision marks the culmination of the surgical performance, leaving patients with a well-orchestrated implantation site.

Postoperative Monitoring and Care:
Following pacemaker implantation, patients are closely monitored in a recovery area. Vital signs are assessed, and the implantation site is inspected for any signs of complications. Patients receive postoperative care instructions, including guidelines for activities, wound care, and medication management. The healthcare team collaborates with patients to ensure a smooth transition into the postoperative phase, fostering healing and optimal recovery.

Recovery and Post-Implantation Care

The completion of pacemaker implantation marks the beginning of a transformative journey toward restored cardiac health. The recovery and post-implantation care phase is crucial for ensuring the optimal functioning of the pacemaker, promoting healing, and empowering individuals to resume their normal activities with newfound rhythm.

Immediate Postoperative Monitoring:
Following pacemaker implantation, individuals are closely monitored in a postoperative recovery area. Vital signs, including heart rate and blood pressure, are assessed to ensure stability. The implantation site is inspected for any signs of bleeding, infection, or other complications. This initial postoperative monitoring is vital for identifying and addressing immediate concerns, setting the stage for a smooth transition into the recovery phase.

Wound Care and Incision Management:
Proper wound care is crucial for promoting optimal healing of the incision site. Patients receive guidance on keeping the incision clean and dry, and healthcare providers may recommend specific practices such as avoiding vigorous scrubbing, using mild soap, and covering the incision with a sterile dressing. Monitoring the incision site for signs of infection, such as redness or swelling, is an integral aspect of post-implantation care.

Activity Guidelines:
While the immediate postoperative period may involve some restrictions, individuals are gradually guided back to their regular activities. Healthcare providers offer specific guidelines regarding physical activity, emphasizing the

importance of avoiding strenuous exercises or heavy lifting during the initial recovery phase. As healing progresses, patients are encouraged to resume their normal routines, with adjustments made based on individual needs and the type of pacemaker implanted.

Medication Management:
Patients often receive specific instructions regarding medications following pacemaker implantation. These may include antibiotics to prevent infection, pain relievers for discomfort, and adjustments to existing medications. It is crucial for individuals to adhere to the prescribed medication regimen and communicate any concerns or side effects to their healthcare providers during the recovery period.

Follow-up Appointments:
Scheduled follow-up appointments play a pivotal role in long-term post-implantation care. These appointments allow healthcare providers to assess the functioning of the pacemaker, check lead stability, and make any necessary adjustments to pacing parameters. Regular monitoring is essential for ensuring the pacemaker continues to meet the individual's cardiac needs and provides an opportunity to address any emerging concerns or questions.

Remote Monitoring:
Advancements in pacemaker technology have

introduced remote monitoring capabilities, allowing healthcare providers to access real-time data from the pacemaker without the need for in-person appointments. Remote monitoring enhances the efficiency of post-implantation care, enabling timely identification of issues, adjustments to pacing parameters, and proactive management of the pacemaker's performance.

Emotional and Psychological Support:
The recovery phase after pacemaker implantation extends beyond physical healing to encompass emotional and psychological well-being. Individuals may experience a range of emotions, including anxiety or adjustment concerns. Healthcare providers, along with support from family and friends, play a vital role in offering emotional support and addressing any psychological aspects of the recovery process.

Lifestyle Adjustments:
Post-implantation care involves considerations for lifestyle adjustments that promote overall cardiac health. Individuals are educated about maintaining a heart-healthy diet, engaging in regular physical activity, managing stress, and avoiding factors that may interfere with pacemaker function. These lifestyle adjustments contribute to the holistic well-being of individuals living with a pacemaker.

Patient Education:

Patient education is an ongoing process that empowers individuals with the knowledge and skills needed to navigate life with a pacemaker successfully. Topics covered may include recognizing signs of potential issues, understanding the importance of follow-up care, and adopting lifestyle choices that support overall cardiovascular health. Education fosters a sense of empowerment, enabling individuals to actively participate in their ongoing care and well-being.

LIVING WITH A PACEMAKER

"I spent a lot of years trying to outrun or outsmart vulnerability by making things certain and definite, black and white, good and bad. My inability to lean into the discomfort of vulnerability limited the fullness of those important experiences that are wrought with uncertainty: Love, belonging, trust, joy, and creativity to name a few."
-Brene Brown

Adjusting to Life with a Pacemaker

The introduction of a pacemaker into one's life marks a significant chapter in the journey toward cardiac health. Adjusting to life with a pacemaker involves more than the physical integration of the device—it encompasses emotional, lifestyle, and psychological adaptations.

Understanding the Pacemaker's Role:
The initial step in adjusting to life with a pacemaker is gaining a comprehensive understanding of the device's role. Individuals, along with their healthcare providers, explore the specifics of the pacemaker implanted, including its type, pacing parameters, and any

additional features. This knowledge forms the foundation for informed decision-making and active participation in one's cardiac care.

Emotional Resilience:
Adjusting to life with a pacemaker often brings forth a range of emotions, including relief, gratitude, and, in some cases, apprehension or anxiety. Recognizing and acknowledging these emotions is crucial for building emotional resilience. Open communication with healthcare providers, support from friends and family, and connecting with others who have undergone a similar journey can contribute to a positive emotional outlook.

Lifestyle Modifications:
Life with a pacemaker may involve certain lifestyle modifications aimed at supporting cardiovascular health. Adopting a heart-healthy diet, engaging in regular physical activity within the parameters set by healthcare providers, and managing stress are integral components. Individuals learn to navigate these adjustments to create a holistic and heart-optimizing lifestyle.

Physical Activity and Exercise:
Individuals with pacemakers can lead active and fulfilling lives, with certain considerations for physical activity. Healthcare providers offer guidelines on exercise intensity and types of activities that are safe and beneficial. This may

involve avoiding activities that could dislodge leads, seeking moderation in vigorous exercises, and maintaining overall cardiovascular fitness.

Pacemaker Checks and Follow-Up:
Regular pacemaker checks and follow-up appointments form an essential part of adapting to life with the device. These appointments allow healthcare providers to monitor the pacemaker's performance, assess lead stability, and make any necessary adjustments to pacing parameters. Consistent follow-up ensures that the pacemaker continues to meet the individual's cardiac needs and provides opportunities for education and support.

Social and Community Support:
Building a network of social and community support plays a pivotal role in the adjustment process. Supportive friends, family, and fellow individuals with pacemakers can provide encouragement, understanding, and shared experiences. Social connections contribute to a sense of community and reduce feelings of isolation, fostering a more positive adjustment to life with a pacemaker.

Travel Considerations:
Life with a pacemaker may include considerations for travel, whether domestic or international. Individuals learn to navigate airport security procedures, carry necessary documentation,

and communicate effectively with healthcare providers to ensure a seamless travel experience. With careful planning, travel becomes an enriching aspect of life rather than a source of concern.

Sexual Activity:
Addressing concerns and questions related to sexual activity is an integral part of adapting to life with a pacemaker. Healthcare providers offer guidance on resuming sexual activity, addressing potential concerns, and ensuring a healthy and fulfilling intimate life. Open communication between partners contributes to a supportive and understanding environment.

Psychological Well-Being:
Psychological well-being is a key component of adjusting to life with a pacemaker. Individuals may engage in mindfulness practices, counseling, or support groups to address any lingering concerns or anxieties. The integration of psychological care into the overall adjustment process promotes a balanced and resilient mental outlook.

Educational Resources:
Access to educational resources plays a crucial role in the adjustment journey. Individuals are encouraged to actively seek information about their specific pacemaker, cardiac health, and lifestyle recommendations. Educational

materials, workshops, and online resources empower individuals to take an active role in their ongoing cardiac care.

Lifestyle Considerations

Pacemaker implantation is a transformative intervention that ensures the heart's rhythm is regulated, allowing individuals to lead active and fulfilling lives. Adjusting to life with a pacemaker involves careful consideration of lifestyle choices to optimize cardiovascular health. This essay explores the various lifestyle considerations after pacemaker implantation, offering insights into how individuals can harmonize their daily routines with the presence of this life-enhancing device.

Physical Activity and Exercise:
Maintaining an active lifestyle is crucial for overall health, and having a pacemaker should not hinder regular physical activity. Healthcare providers guide individuals on the types and intensity of exercises that are safe and beneficial. Generally, activities like walking, cycling, and swimming are encouraged, while contact sports or activities that involve a risk of falls may be limited. Regular exercise contributes to cardiovascular fitness, enhances mood, and supports overall well-being.

Dietary Choices:

A heart-healthy diet is paramount for individuals with pacemakers. Reducing sodium intake helps manage blood pressure, while incorporating a variety of fruits, vegetables, whole grains, and lean proteins contributes to overall cardiovascular health. Healthcare providers may offer specific dietary guidelines based on individual health needs and may recommend adjustments to accommodate any medication requirements.

Stress Management:
Managing stress is essential for cardiovascular health. Individuals with pacemakers are encouraged to adopt stress-reducing practices such as mindfulness, meditation, yoga, or deep-breathing exercises. Finding effective coping mechanisms not only supports emotional well-being but also contributes to a harmonious and balanced lifestyle.

Hydration and Caffeine Intake:
Adequate hydration is important for overall health, but individuals with pacemakers should be mindful of their fluid intake. Consuming moderate amounts of caffeine is generally considered safe, but excessive intake may be discouraged, as it can potentially affect heart rhythm. Balancing hydration and caffeine consumption contributes to maintaining optimal pacemaker function.

Alcohol Consumption:

Moderate alcohol consumption is generally considered acceptable for individuals with pacemakers. However, excessive alcohol intake can have adverse effects on cardiovascular health and may interact with medications. It is important for individuals to discuss their alcohol consumption with healthcare providers, who can offer personalized guidance based on individual health factors.

Sleep Hygiene:
Quality sleep is crucial for overall health and well-being. Individuals with pacemakers should prioritize good sleep hygiene, including maintaining a consistent sleep schedule, creating a comfortable sleep environment, and avoiding excessive caffeine intake close to bedtime. Adequate and restful sleep supports optimal cardiovascular function and overall vitality.

Travel Considerations:
Individuals with pacemakers can enjoy travel, but some considerations are necessary. Informing airport security about the presence of the pacemaker, carrying necessary documentation, and avoiding prolonged exposure to metal detectors are important. Individuals should also be aware of the availability of medical facilities at their travel destination and plan accordingly.

Regular Pacemaker Checks and Follow-Up:
Scheduled pacemaker checks and follow-

up appointments are integral to lifestyle considerations. Regular monitoring ensures that the pacemaker functions optimally and allows healthcare providers to make any necessary adjustments to pacing parameters. Consistent follow-up contributes to the overall management of cardiovascular health and provides an opportunity for ongoing education and support.

Sexual Activity:
Addressing concerns and questions related to sexual activity is a crucial aspect of lifestyle considerations after pacemaker implantation. In most cases, individuals can resume sexual activity after the initial recovery period. Open communication between partners, along with guidance from healthcare providers, contributes to a healthy and fulfilling intimate life.

Psychological Well-Being:
Maintaining psychological well-being is a key component of lifestyle considerations. Individuals may experience a range of emotions after pacemaker implantation, and seeking support through counseling, support groups, or other mental health resources can be beneficial. A positive mental outlook contributes to overall well-being and enhances the adaptation to life with a pacemaker.

Educational Resources and Support:
Access to educational resources and support is

essential for individuals adjusting to life with a pacemaker. Educational materials, workshops, and online resources provide information about the specific pacemaker, lifestyle recommendations, and ongoing cardiac care. Building a network of support, including friends, family, and fellow individuals with pacemakers, fosters a sense of community and understanding.

Dietary Guidelines

Diet plays a pivotal role in maintaining overall health and supporting cardiovascular function. After pacemaker implantation, individuals often seek guidance on dietary choices that promote well-being and complement the optimal functioning of the device. This text explores dietary guidelines tailored for individuals with pacemakers, emphasizing the importance of nourishing the body while harmonizing with the rhythms of cardiovascular health.

Balancing Sodium Intake:
Managing sodium intake is crucial for individuals with pacemakers, especially those dealing with conditions such as hypertension. High sodium levels can contribute to elevated blood pressure, potentially impacting cardiovascular health. Therefore, it is advisable to limit the consumption of processed and salty foods, opting for fresh fruits, vegetables, whole grains, and lean proteins

instead.

Hydration and Fluid Intake:
Adequate hydration is essential for overall health, but individuals with pacemakers should be mindful of their fluid intake. While staying hydrated is important, excessive fluid consumption can lead to increased stress on the heart. Striking a balance by maintaining proper hydration without overloading the cardiovascular system is key.

Heart-Healthy Fats:
Incorporating heart-healthy fats into the diet is beneficial for cardiovascular health. Omega-3 fatty acids, found in fatty fish, flaxseeds, and walnuts, have been associated with positive heart outcomes. Olive oil, avocados, and nuts are sources of monounsaturated fats that contribute to a heart-healthy diet. These fats help maintain optimal cholesterol levels, supporting cardiovascular well-being.

Lean Proteins:
Choosing lean protein sources is essential for individuals with pacemakers. Poultry, fish, legumes, and plant-based proteins are preferable over processed and fatty meats. Lean proteins provide essential amino acids without the saturated fat content that may contribute to heart-related issues.

High-Fiber Foods:

A diet rich in fiber offers numerous benefits for cardiovascular health. High-fiber foods, including fruits, vegetables, whole grains, and legumes, help maintain healthy cholesterol levels, regulate blood sugar, and support digestive health. These dietary components contribute to an overall heart-healthy lifestyle.

Limiting Caffeine and Alcohol:
While moderate caffeine consumption is generally considered safe, excessive intake may have stimulant effects on the heart, potentially impacting rhythm. Similarly, individuals with pacemakers are advised to limit alcohol consumption. Both caffeine and alcohol should be enjoyed in moderation, with individuals paying attention to their body's responses and consulting with healthcare providers as needed.

Avoiding Excessive Sugar and Processed Foods:
Excessive sugar intake and consumption of processed foods are associated with various health issues, including obesity and diabetes, which can affect cardiovascular health. Individuals with pacemakers are encouraged to limit their intake of sugary beverages, candies, and highly processed foods. Opting for whole, nutrient-dense foods supports overall well-being.

Individualized Dietary Plans:
Dietary needs vary among individuals, and personalized dietary plans can optimize

health outcomes after pacemaker implantation. Healthcare providers, including registered dietitians, can offer individualized guidance based on factors such as age, weight, medical history, and specific health goals. Customized plans ensure that dietary recommendations align with the unique needs of each individual.

Monitoring Electrolyte Levels:
Pacemakers regulate heart rhythm by managing the flow of electrical impulses. Monitoring electrolyte levels, including potassium and magnesium, is crucial for maintaining the proper functioning of the device. Foods rich in potassium, such as bananas, oranges, and leafy greens, contribute to electrolyte balance and support heart health.

Supplements and Medication Interaction:
Individuals with pacemakers may be prescribed medications or supplements to manage specific health conditions. It is essential to communicate openly with healthcare providers about any dietary supplements or over-the-counter medications being taken, as these can interact with prescribed medications or impact overall health.

Exercise Guidelines

Exercise is a cornerstone of a healthy lifestyle, contributing to overall well-being and cardiovascular health. After pacemaker implantation, individuals often wonder about the appropriate guidelines for physical activity.

Consultation with Healthcare Providers:
Before engaging in any exercise program after pacemaker implantation, it is crucial to consult with healthcare providers. Cardiologists and other medical professionals will assess individual health status, the type of pacemaker implanted, and specific cardiac considerations to provide personalized exercise recommendations. This initial consultation lays the foundation for a safe and effective exercise plan.

Gradual Return to Exercise:
After pacemaker implantation, individuals may need to make a gradual return to exercise, especially if they have been sedentary or experienced limitations prior to the procedure. Starting with low-impact activities such as walking or stationary cycling allows the body to adapt gradually and minimizes the risk of complications.

Aerobic Exercise:
Aerobic exercise, also known as cardiovascular or endurance exercise, is beneficial for heart health. Individuals with pacemakers can engage in aerobic activities such as walking, jogging, cycling, swimming, and dancing. These activities help improve cardiovascular fitness, enhance

circulation, and contribute to overall well-being.

Resistance Training:
Resistance training, involving the use of weights or resistance bands, is generally safe for individuals with pacemakers. Strength training exercises help build and maintain muscle mass, supporting overall physical function. It is essential to start with light weights and gradually progress, ensuring proper form to avoid strain.

Flexibility and Stretching:
Incorporating flexibility and stretching exercises into the routine promotes joint health and flexibility. Gentle stretching helps improve range of motion, reduces the risk of injuries, and contributes to overall physical comfort. Yoga and tai chi are examples of activities that combine flexibility, balance, and relaxation.

Avoiding High-Risk Activities:
While regular exercise is encouraged, individuals with pacemakers should avoid certain high-risk activities that may pose a danger to the device or overall health. Activities such as contact sports, high-impact activities, and exercises that involve sudden, jerky movements should be approached with caution or avoided altogether.

Listening to the Body:
Listening to the body's signals is essential during and after exercise. Individuals should be attentive to any discomfort, pain, dizziness, or unusual

symptoms during physical activity. If such symptoms occur, it is crucial to stop the activity and consult with healthcare providers to ensure proper evaluation and adjustments to the exercise plan.

Hydration and Temperature Considerations:
Proper hydration is important during exercise, and individuals with pacemakers should pay attention to their fluid intake. Additionally, exercising in extreme temperatures, whether excessively hot or cold, may affect cardiovascular function. Staying hydrated and adjusting the exercise environment to moderate temperatures contribute to a safe and enjoyable exercise experience.

Regular Monitoring and Follow-Up:
Regular monitoring of exercise intensity and duration is essential, especially in the initial phases after pacemaker implantation. Follow-up appointments with healthcare providers allow for ongoing assessment, adjustments to exercise plans, and addressing any concerns or questions related to physical activity.

Individualized Exercise Plans:
Exercise plans should be individualized based on factors such as age, fitness level, overall health, and the type of pacemaker implanted. Tailoring exercise recommendations to the specific needs of each individual ensures that the benefits of

physical activity are maximized while minimizing potential risks.

Educational Resources and Support:
Access to educational resources and support is valuable for individuals navigating exercise after pacemaker implantation. Information about safe exercise practices, guidelines for specific activities, and insights from healthcare professionals contribute to a well-informed and confident approach to physical activity.

REMOTE MONITORING AND FOLLOWUP CARE

"I couldn't find the remote control to the remote control."
-Steven Wright

Importance of Regular Followup

The journey towards optimal cardiovascular health does not conclude with the implantation procedure. Regular follow-up appointments with healthcare providers play a pivotal role in ensuring the continued efficacy and well-being of individuals with pacemakers.

Monitoring Pacemaker Function:
Regular follow-up appointments are essential for monitoring the functionality of the pacemaker. During these appointments, healthcare providers assess the device's performance, ensuring that it continues to regulate the heart's rhythm effectively. Parameters such as pacing thresholds, lead impedance, and battery status are routinely checked to identify any deviations from the expected values, allowing for timely interventions

if needed.

Adjusting Pacing Parameters:
The individualized nature of pacemaker settings necessitates periodic adjustments to pacing parameters. Follow-up appointments provide healthcare providers with the opportunity to fine-tune these settings based on the individual's evolving health status. Optimizing pacing parameters ensures that the pacemaker adapts to the dynamic needs of the heart, promoting optimal cardiac function.

Lead Stability Assessment:
The stability of the leads, which are the thin wires connecting the pacemaker to the heart, is a critical aspect of long-term pacemaker performance. Regular follow-up appointments include assessments of lead stability through imaging techniques such as fluoroscopy. Identifying and addressing any issues related to lead dislodgment or malfunction is crucial for maintaining the device's efficacy.

Battery Life Monitoring:
Pacemaker batteries have a limited lifespan, typically ranging from 5 to 15 years depending on factors such as device type and usage. Regular follow-up appointments involve monitoring the pacemaker's battery life, allowing healthcare providers to predict when a battery replacement may be necessary. This proactive approach ensures

that the replacement is performed before the battery is depleted, preventing potential device failure.

Detecting and Addressing Complications:
While pacemaker implantation is generally a safe procedure, complications may arise over time. Regular follow-up appointments provide a platform for healthcare providers to detect and address any complications promptly. Common complications may include infections, lead-related issues, or device-related discomfort. Early identification and intervention contribute to minimizing the impact of complications on the individual's health.

Medication Management and Adjustment:
Individuals with pacemakers may be prescribed medications to manage underlying cardiac conditions. Regular follow-up appointments allow healthcare providers to assess the ongoing need for medications, adjust dosages as necessary, and address any side effects. Medication management is an integral component of overall cardiac care, contributing to the optimization of cardiovascular health.

Evaluation of Overall Cardiovascular Health:
Beyond pacemaker-specific assessments, regular follow-up appointments provide an opportunity to evaluate the individual's overall cardiovascular health. Healthcare providers may monitor

blood pressure, assess cholesterol levels, and address lifestyle factors that influence heart health. This holistic approach ensures that the individual receives comprehensive care, promoting cardiovascular well-being beyond pacemaker management.

Education and Support:
Regular follow-up appointments serve as valuable opportunities for patient education and support. Healthcare providers can offer guidance on lifestyle modifications, answer questions, and address any concerns or anxieties individuals may have about living with a pacemaker. Empowering individuals with knowledge fosters active participation in their own health and well-being.

Psychosocial Support and Mental Health:
Living with a pacemaker can impact an individual's psychosocial well-being. Regular follow-up appointments provide a platform for healthcare providers to address the emotional and psychological aspects of life with a pacemaker. Supportive discussions, counseling, and access to mental health resources contribute to a holistic approach that nurtures both the physical and emotional dimensions of heart health.

Promoting Long-Term Compliance:
Regular follow-up appointments contribute to the establishment of a long-term relationship

between individuals and their healthcare providers. This ongoing connection fosters trust, communication, and a sense of partnership in managing cardiovascular health. Promoting long-term compliance with follow-up recommendations ensures that individuals remain actively engaged in their cardiac care.

Remote Monitoring Technology

Advancements in medical technology have brought about transformative changes in the way healthcare is delivered, particularly in the field of cardiology. Remote monitoring technology for pacemakers represents a groundbreaking development, offering a paradigm shift in the management and care of individuals with cardiac rhythm disorders.

Evolution of Remote Monitoring:
Traditionally, the monitoring of pacemakers required individuals to visit healthcare facilities for periodic check-ups, during which healthcare providers would assess the device's performance, make necessary adjustments, and address any emerging issues. The introduction of remote monitoring technology marks a significant departure from this model, allowing for real-time data collection and analysis without the need for in-person visits.

Functionality of Remote Monitoring:
Remote monitoring technology for pacemakers involves the use of wireless communication systems to transmit data from the implanted device to a secure remote server. This data includes information about the pacemaker's functioning, such as pacing thresholds, battery status, lead impedance, and arrhythmia events. The technology enables healthcare providers to access this information remotely, facilitating timely and proactive management of the pacemaker.

Continuous Surveillance and Timely Intervention:
One of the key advantages of remote monitoring is the ability to provide continuous surveillance of the pacemaker's performance. Real-time data transmission allows healthcare providers to promptly identify any deviations from the expected parameters. This enables timely intervention, reducing the risk of complications and ensuring that the pacemaker continues to meet the individual's cardiac needs.

Early Detection of Issues and Complications:
Remote monitoring technology enhances the early detection of potential issues and complications related to pacemaker function. Changes in pacing thresholds, lead stability, or other parameters can be identified promptly, allowing healthcare providers to address these

issues before they escalate. This proactive approach contributes to improved patient outcomes and a reduced likelihood of emergency interventions.

Enhanced Patient Convenience and Compliance:
For individuals with pacemakers, remote monitoring offers enhanced convenience and increased compliance with follow-up care. The need for frequent in-person visits is significantly reduced, and individuals can go about their daily lives with the assurance that their pacemaker is being continuously monitored. This convenience encourages better adherence to recommended follow-up schedules, contributing to overall cardiovascular health.

Reduced Healthcare Costs:
Remote monitoring technology has the potential to reduce healthcare costs associated with traditional in-person follow-up appointments. By minimizing the need for physical visits and enabling early intervention, the technology can lead to more efficient use of healthcare resources. Additionally, the proactive management of pacemakers through remote monitoring may contribute to preventing costly emergency interventions.

Integration of Artificial Intelligence (AI) and Predictive Analytics:
The integration of artificial intelligence (AI)

and predictive analytics further enhances the capabilities of remote monitoring technology. AI algorithms can analyze vast amounts of data, identify patterns, and predict potential issues with pacemaker function. This predictive capability allows healthcare providers to intervene even before abnormalities become clinically apparent, ushering in a new era of precision medicine.

Data Security and Patient Privacy:
Given the sensitive nature of health data, ensuring robust security and patient privacy is paramount in remote monitoring technology. Advanced encryption methods and secure communication protocols are implemented to safeguard the transmission and storage of patient information. Strict adherence to healthcare data protection regulations ensures that patient privacy remains a top priority in the deployment of remote monitoring systems.

Patient Education and Empowerment:
Remote monitoring technology not only enhances the surveillance and management of pacemakers but also plays a role in patient education and empowerment. Individuals can gain insights into their own health data through patient portals, fostering a sense of engagement and active participation in their cardiac care. Education about interpreting remote monitoring data empowers individuals to be proactive in

maintaining their cardiovascular health.

Future Implications and Potential Developments:
The evolution of remote monitoring technology for pacemakers opens the door to exciting possibilities for future developments. Continuous advancements in AI, machine learning, and sensor technologies may further refine the capabilities of remote monitoring systems. The integration of data from wearable devices and other health metrics could provide a comprehensive overview of an individual's overall health, contributing to a more holistic approach to cardiac care.

Typical Followup Schedule

Following the procedure, a structured and comprehensive follow-up schedule becomes a lifeline of care, monitoring the pacemaker's performance, addressing emerging issues, and supporting overall cardiovascular health.

Immediate Post-Implantation Period:
The immediate post-implantation period involves close monitoring to assess the patient's recovery and ensure the pacemaker is functioning as expected. This may include an overnight hospital stay for observation, during which healthcare providers monitor vital signs, assess wound healing, and confirm the proper functioning of the pacemaker.

First Follow-Up Appointment (1-2 Weeks):
The first follow-up appointment typically occurs within the first one to two weeks after pacemaker implantation. This initial visit allows healthcare providers to assess the incision site, address any immediate concerns or discomfort, and perform a preliminary check of the pacemaker's settings. It serves as a crucial step in ensuring a smooth transition from the implantation procedure to ongoing care.

Second Follow-Up Appointment (4-6 Weeks):
The second follow-up appointment, scheduled around four to six weeks post-implantation, involves a more comprehensive assessment of the pacemaker's performance. Healthcare providers conduct a thorough check of pacing parameters, assess lead stability, and address any concerns or questions the patient may have. This visit serves as an important checkpoint to ensure the pacemaker is adapting well to the individual's physiological needs.

Subsequent Follow-Up Appointments (Every 3-12 Months):
Following the initial post-implantation period, individuals with pacemakers enter into a regular follow-up schedule, which may occur every three to twelve months, depending on the individual's health status and the healthcare provider's recommendations. These appointments involve

a systematic evaluation of the pacemaker's functioning, lead stability, battery life, and overall cardiovascular health.

Remote Monitoring and Telehealth Visits:
Advancements in technology have introduced remote monitoring capabilities, allowing healthcare providers to access real-time data from the pacemaker without the need for in-person visits. Remote monitoring is often complemented by occasional telehealth visits, providing an opportunity for healthcare providers and patients to discuss any concerns, review data, and make necessary adjustments to pacing parameters.

Annual Comprehensive Evaluations:
At least once a year, individuals with pacemakers typically undergo a more comprehensive evaluation, which may include additional diagnostic tests such as electrocardiograms (ECGs), echocardiograms, or stress tests. These annual assessments provide a more in-depth understanding of the individual's overall cardiovascular health and help guide long-term management strategies.

Battery Replacement Planning (Approximately Every 5-15 Years):
Pacemaker batteries have a limited lifespan, generally ranging from 5 to 15 years, depending on factors such as device type and usage. As the battery approaches the end of its

life, healthcare providers plan for a battery replacement procedure. This involves a scheduled outpatient visit during which the old generator is replaced with a new one, ensuring continuous and uninterrupted pacing.

Individualized Follow-Up Plans:
The follow-up schedule is highly individualized based on factors such as age, overall health, the specific pacemaker implanted, and any underlying cardiac conditions. Healthcare providers tailor the frequency and nature of follow-up appointments to meet the unique needs of each individual, ensuring that the pacemaker remains optimized for their specific physiological requirements.

Patient Education and Empowerment:
Throughout the follow-up schedule, patient education plays a crucial role. Healthcare providers use these appointments as opportunities to educate individuals about their pacemakers, heart health, and lifestyle considerations. Empowering individuals with knowledge fosters active participation in their cardiac care, enabling them to make informed decisions and manage their well-being effectively.

Psychosocial Support:
In addition to the technical assessments, follow-up appointments also serve as opportunities for psychosocial support. Living with a pacemaker may impact an individual's emotional well-

being, and healthcare providers use these visits to address any concerns, provide counseling if needed, and foster a supportive environment that nurtures both physical and mental health.

COMMON ISSUES AND CONCERNS

"There were complications, there were questions; but they were so much more together than they were anything else."
— Henry James

Managing Pain and Discomfort

While the benefits are significant, individuals may experience varying degrees of pain and discomfort during the recovery period.

Understanding Post-Implantation Pain:
Pain and discomfort after pacemaker implantation are common, given that the procedure involves making an incision to insert the device beneath the skin, typically in the chest area. The level of pain can vary among individuals, influenced by factors such as pain tolerance, overall health, and the complexity of the implantation.

Immediate Post-Operative Care:
In the immediate post-operative period, individuals are closely monitored for

pain management. Healthcare providers may administer pain medications, such as acetaminophen or nonsteroidal anti-inflammatory drugs (NSAIDs), to alleviate discomfort. Opioid medications may be prescribed for more severe pain but are typically used judiciously due to the potential for side effects and dependency.

Pain Management Medications:
Following discharge, individuals may continue with prescribed pain medications to manage discomfort. It is crucial to adhere to the recommended dosage and frequency as directed by healthcare providers. Consistent and responsible use of pain management medications helps individuals strike a balance between alleviating discomfort and minimizing potential side effects.

Application of Ice Packs:
Ice packs can be applied to the incision site to help reduce swelling and numb the area, providing relief from localized pain. It is essential to use a cloth or towel to wrap the ice pack and avoid direct skin contact to prevent frostbite. The intermittent application of ice in the initial days post-implantation can contribute to enhanced comfort.

Elevating the Arm:
As the pacemaker is often implanted near the shoulder area, elevating the arm on the side of

the implant can help reduce strain on the incision site. Keeping the arm elevated, especially during periods of rest, can alleviate discomfort and promote optimal healing. This simple yet effective measure aids in minimizing pain associated with movement.

Deep Breathing and Relaxation Techniques:
Deep breathing exercises and relaxation techniques can be beneficial in managing post-implantation discomfort. Controlled, slow, and deep breaths can help relax the body and alleviate tension. Engaging in practices such as meditation or guided imagery can also contribute to a sense of calm, reducing overall perceived pain.

Gradual Resumption of Activities:
While rest is essential for recovery, gradually resuming light activities can contribute to improved circulation and reduced stiffness. Healthcare providers typically provide guidelines on the gradual resumption of daily activities, avoiding strenuous movements or lifting heavy objects during the initial recovery phase.

Wound Care and Hygiene:
Proper wound care and hygiene are critical for preventing infection and minimizing discomfort. Keeping the incision site clean, dry, and free from irritation supports optimal healing. Individuals should follow healthcare providers' instructions regarding showering, dressing changes, and

avoiding activities that may compromise the incision site.

Communication with Healthcare Providers:
Open and transparent communication with healthcare providers is crucial during the recovery period. Individuals should not hesitate to discuss their pain levels, concerns, or any unexpected symptoms with their healthcare team. This communication allows for timely adjustments to the pain management plan and ensures that individual needs are addressed effectively.

Psychosocial Support:
Pain and discomfort after pacemaker implantation can have psychosocial implications. Seeking support from friends, family, or support groups can provide emotional reassurance during the recovery process. Psychosocial support is an integral component of holistic care, addressing both the physical and emotional aspects of post-implantation recovery.

Individualized Pain Management Plans:
Recognizing that individuals may have unique pain experiences, healthcare providers work collaboratively with patients to develop individualized pain management plans. These plans take into account factors such as pre-existing health conditions, medication sensitivities, and personal preferences, ensuring a tailored approach to managing post-implantation

discomfort.

Recognizing and Addressing Complications

Individuals may occasionally experience complications related to the device. Recognizing and promptly addressing these complications are crucial aspects of ensuring the ongoing well-being of individuals with pacemakers.

Common Complications and Their Causes:
1. Infection: Infections at the implantation site are potential complications. Bacterial contamination during the procedure, poor wound care, or underlying medical conditions can contribute to infections.

2. Lead Dislodgment or Fracture: The leads, which connect the pacemaker to the heart, may become dislodged or fractured, affecting the device's ability to regulate heart rhythm. Trauma, repetitive movement, or lead fatigue over time can contribute to this complication.

3. Pneumothorax: During pacemaker implantation, the puncture of the lung lining may lead to pneumothorax, causing air to accumulate between the lung and chest wall. This can result in breathing difficulties and discomfort.

4. Hematoma: Accumulation of blood at the

implantation site can lead to a hematoma. Excessive bleeding during the procedure or poor blood clotting can contribute to hematoma formation.

5. Thrombosis: Blood clots may form on the leads or within the veins, potentially leading to complications such as pulmonary embolism or device malfunction. Factors like blood clotting disorders or inadequate anticoagulation therapy can contribute to thrombosis.

6. Device Malfunction: Technical issues with the pacemaker itself, such as battery depletion, lead failure, or software malfunctions, can compromise its performance and effectiveness in regulating heart rhythm.

Early Signs and Symptoms:
Recognizing early signs and symptoms of complications is crucial for prompt intervention. These may include:
- Fever or localized warmth: Indicative of infection.
- Swelling, redness, or tenderness at the implantation site: Suggestive of hematoma or infection.
- Changes in heart rate or rhythm: Potential signs of lead dislodgment or device malfunction.
- Shortness of breath or chest pain: Indicative of pneumothorax or thrombosis.

Diagnostic Tools and Imaging:

Healthcare providers employ various diagnostic tools and imaging techniques to assess and confirm complications. These may include:
- Chest X-rays: Useful for identifying pneumothorax, lead position, and signs of heart failure.
- Echocardiograms: Provide detailed images of the heart and can detect issues such as lead dislodgment or thrombosis.
- Electrophysiological Studies: Assess the electrical activity of the heart, aiding in the identification of arrhythmias or lead-related complications.

Strategies for Timely Intervention:
1. Regular Follow-Up Appointments: Scheduled follow-up appointments allow healthcare providers to monitor the pacemaker's performance and address emerging issues before they escalate.

2. Remote Monitoring Technology: Utilizing remote monitoring technology enables real-time data transmission, allowing healthcare providers to detect and address potential complications promptly.

3. Patient Education: Educating individuals about the signs and symptoms of complications empowers them to seek timely medical attention. Clear communication channels between healthcare providers and patients foster a proactive approach to cardiac health.

4. Early Intervention Protocols: Establishing protocols for early intervention in the event of complications ensures that healthcare providers can swiftly address emerging issues, minimizing the impact on the individual's well-being.

5. Collaborative Approach: A collaborative approach involving cardiologists, electrophysiologists, and other healthcare professionals ensures comprehensive care and timely interventions in the face of complications.

6. Individualized Care Plans: Recognizing that complications can vary among individuals, healthcare providers develop individualized care plans based on factors such as age, overall health, and the nature of the complication.

Psychosocial Support:
Experiencing complications with a pacemaker can be emotionally challenging. Psychosocial support, including counseling and support groups, plays a vital role in helping individuals cope with the emotional aspects of complications, fostering resilience and well-being.

Troubleshooting Guide for Patients and Caregivers

This troubleshooting guide is designed to empower patients and caregivers with the knowledge and understanding needed to navigate common challenges, ensuring the optimal functioning of the pacemaker and supporting the well-being of individuals relying on these life-enhancing devices.

Understanding the Pacemaker:
Before delving into troubleshooting, it's essential to have a basic understanding of how a pacemaker works. A pacemaker is a small, implanted device that regulates the heart's rhythm by sending electrical signals to the heart muscles. It consists of a generator (containing the battery and electronic circuits) and leads (thin wires connecting the generator to the heart).

Common Issues and Troubleshooting Steps:

1. Change in Symptoms or Feeling Unwell:
   - Troubleshooting Steps:
   - Pay attention to any changes in symptoms, such as dizziness, fatigue, or shortness of breath.
   - Check if there are any signs of infection, redness, or swelling around the pacemaker site.
   - Contact healthcare providers promptly if symptoms persist or worsen.

2. Feeling a Strong or Irregular Heartbeat:
   - Troubleshooting Steps:
   - Relax and take a few deep breaths to ensure calmness.
   - Avoid stimulants like caffeine or nicotine.
   - If symptoms persist, contact healthcare providers for an evaluation.

3. Skin Redness, Swelling, or Warmth at the Implantation Site:
   - Troubleshooting Steps:
     - Ensure proper wound care and hygiene.
     - Monitor for signs of infection, such as fever.
   - Contact healthcare providers if redness, swelling, or warmth persists or worsens.

4. Change in Exercise Tolerance or Physical Activity Levels:
   - Troubleshooting Steps:
   - Gradually resume physical activities as advised by healthcare providers.
   - Communicate any unusual symptoms or discomfort during exercise.
   - Seek guidance on appropriate exercise levels and modifications if needed.

5. Device Alarms or Beeping Sounds:
   - Troubleshooting Steps:
   - Refer to the pacemaker identification card for information on device type and manufacturer.
   - Contact the device clinic or healthcare providers immediately if the device emits alarms or unusual sounds.

6. Unexplained Fatigue or Weakness:
   - Troubleshooting Steps:
   - Ensure adequate rest and sleep.
   - Check for any signs of anemia or other underlying health issues.
   - Report persistent fatigue or weakness to

healthcare providers.

7. Remote Monitoring Alerts:
   - Troubleshooting Steps:
      - Follow instructions provided by the remote monitoring system.
      - Contact healthcare providers promptly if there are concerns or if the alerts indicate a potential issue.

8. Chest Pain or Discomfort:
   - Troubleshooting Steps:
      - Assess the nature and duration of chest pain.
      - Seek immediate medical attention if chest pain is severe, prolonged, or accompanied by other concerning symptoms.

When to Seek Professional Help:
While this guide provides general troubleshooting steps, it's crucial to recognize situations that warrant immediate professional assistance. Seek prompt medical attention if experiencing:
- Severe or persistent chest pain.
- Unexplained fainting or loss of consciousness.
- Difficulty breathing.
- Device alarms or sounds indicating a critical issue.
- Signs of infection, such as fever, increasing redness, or discharge at the implantation site.

The Role of Regular Follow-Up Appointments:
Regular follow-up appointments with healthcare providers are integral to the ongoing

care of individuals with pacemakers. These appointments allow for comprehensive device checks, adjustments to pacing parameters, and the identification of potential issues before they become critical. Adhering to scheduled follow-up visits ensures proactive management of the pacemaker's performance and contributes to long-term cardiac health.

Living with a pacemaker involves an active partnership between individuals, caregivers, and healthcare providers. By understanding common issues and following appropriate troubleshooting steps, individuals and their caregivers can contribute to the optimal functioning of the pacemaker and overall well-being.

EMOTIONAL AND PSYCHOLOGICAL CONSIDERATIONS

"Nothing but the chance to say, wordlessly, Here; you've been carrying that alone for a long time. Let me carry it with you awhile."
—*Julie Berry*

Coping with the Emotional Impact

Individuals with pacemakers and their caregivers may navigate a range of emotions as they adapt to life with this life-enhancing device. This text explores the emotional impact of living with a pacemaker and offers strategies for coping with these sentiments, fostering resilience, and embracing a fulfilling life.

Understanding the Emotional Landscape:
Receiving a pacemaker is often a life-changing event, and individuals may experience a spectrum of emotions in response to this significant transition. Common emotional responses include:
- Anxiety and Fear: Concerns about the unknown, the implantation procedure, or potential

complications can lead to heightened anxiety.

- Grief or Loss: Adjusting to life with a pacemaker may entail a sense of loss of normalcy or the perception of one's body changing.

- Depression: Coping with a chronic condition can sometimes lead to feelings of sadness or depression.

- Anger or Frustration: Individuals may feel frustration or anger at the need for medical intervention or the perceived limitations imposed by the pacemaker.

Coping Strategies for Emotional Well-being:

1. Education and Information:
   - Strategy:
   - Understanding the pacemaker, its purpose, and the associated procedures can demystify the experience, alleviating anxiety and fear.
   - Engage in open communication with healthcare providers to address any lingering questions or concerns.

2. Peer Support and Sharing Experiences:
   - Strategy:
   - Connect with support groups or individuals who have experienced similar journeys with pacemakers.
   - Sharing experiences and insights fosters a sense of community and reduces feelings of isolation.

3. Embracing a Positive Mindset:

- Strategy:

- Focus on the positive aspects of life with a pacemaker, such as improved health and the ability to engage in meaningful activities.

- Cultivate gratitude for the advancements in medical technology that enable a fuller life.

4. Professional Counseling:
- Strategy:

- Seek the guidance of a mental health professional or counselor to navigate complex emotions.

- Counseling provides a safe space to explore and address underlying feelings, promoting emotional well-being.

5. Setting Realistic Expectations:
- Strategy:

- Establish realistic expectations for daily activities, acknowledging that adjustments may be needed.

- Celebrate personal milestones and achievements, no matter how small, to cultivate a positive outlook.

6. Engaging in Physical Activity:
- Strategy:

- Physical activity, within the limits recommended by healthcare providers, contributes to both physical and emotional well-being.

- Exercise releases endorphins, which can

positively impact mood and reduce stress.

7. Open Communication with Loved Ones:
   - Strategy:
   - Communicate openly with family and friends about emotional experiences and needs.
   - Establishing a support system allows loved ones to provide understanding and encouragement.

8. Mindfulness and Relaxation Techniques:
   - Strategy:
   - Practice mindfulness and relaxation techniques, such as meditation or deep breathing exercises.
   - These techniques can help manage stress, promote a sense of calm, and enhance overall emotional resilience.

9. Participation in Hobbies and Activities:
   - Strategy:
   - Engaging in hobbies and activities that bring joy and fulfillment fosters a sense of purpose.
   - Pursuing interests contributes to a balanced and meaningful life beyond the context of the pacemaker.

10. Regular Check-ins with Healthcare Providers:
   - Strategy:
   - Regular follow-up appointments provide an opportunity to discuss emotional well-being with healthcare providers.
   - Open communication ensures that

emotional concerns are addressed as an integral part of overall care.

Addressing Caregiver and Family Dynamics:

Living with a pacemaker not only affects the individual directly but also has implications for caregivers and family members. Strategies for addressing the emotional impact on caregivers and family include:

- Open Communication: Foster open communication within the family to share feelings, concerns, and expectations.
- Educational Support: Ensure that caregivers have access to educational resources and information about the pacemaker to alleviate concerns.
- Respite and Self-Care: Encourage caregivers to prioritize self-care and seek respite when needed to prevent burnout.
- Family Support Systems: Build a support network within the family, allowing for mutual understanding and collaboration in managing emotional aspects.

Support Systems for Patients and Caregivers

Living with a pacemaker is not only a personal journey but also a shared experience that extends to the support systems surrounding individuals with cardiac rhythm disorders. Both patients and caregivers play crucial roles in adapting to life with a pacemaker, and a robust support system enhances the overall well-being of those involved.

The Significance of Support Systems:
Support systems are integral components of the holistic care framework for individuals living with a pacemaker. These systems encompass various layers, including family, friends, healthcare providers, and support groups. They serve as pillars of strength, providing emotional, practical, and informational support to navigate the challenges associated with cardiac health and pacemaker management.

Roles of Patients in Building Support Systems:

1. Open Communication:
   - Role:
   - Patients play a key role in fostering open communication within their support systems.
   - Sharing experiences, concerns, and needs with loved ones allows for a deeper understanding of the individual's journey.

2. Education and Awareness:
   - Role:
   - Patients contribute to building a supportive environment by educating their support network about pacemakers.
   - Providing information about the device, its purpose, and potential challenges fosters awareness and dispels misconceptions.

3. Setting Boundaries and Expressing Needs:
- Role:

- Clearly expressing personal boundaries and needs allows patients to receive support tailored to their preferences.

- Open communication about limitations and expectations fosters a supportive atmosphere.

4. Active Participation in Support Groups:
- Role:

- Joining support groups or online communities enables patients to connect with others facing similar experiences.

- Active participation fosters a sense of community, shared knowledge, and mutual encouragement.

5. Advocating for Self-Care:
- Role:

- Patients play a crucial role in advocating for their own self-care and well-being.

- Communicating the importance of rest, regular exercise, and adherence to healthcare recommendations contributes to long-term health.

Roles of Caregivers in Building Support Systems:

1. Emotional Support:
- Role:

- Caregivers provide emotional support by actively listening, offering reassurance, and acknowledging the challenges patients may face.

- Creating a compassionate and understanding environment is essential for the emotional well-being of both the patient and the caregiver.

2. Practical Assistance:
  - Role:
  - Caregivers assist with practical tasks, such as accompanying patients to medical appointments, helping with daily activities, and providing transportation.
  - Offering practical assistance alleviates the burden on patients and fosters a sense of partnership in managing health.

3. Educational Empowerment:
  - Role:
  - Caregivers actively engage in learning about pacemakers, their function, and potential challenges.
  - Being informed empowers caregivers to provide better support and effectively collaborate with healthcare providers.

4. Advocacy for Healthcare Needs:
  - Role:
  - Caregivers act as advocates for the healthcare needs of the patient.
  - Collaborating with healthcare providers, scheduling appointments, and ensuring medication adherence are integral aspects of caregiving.

5. Resilience and Adaptability:
   - Role:
   - Caregivers demonstrate resilience and adaptability in the face of challenges.
   - Maintaining a positive outlook, being flexible, and supporting the patient through adjustments contribute to a healthier and more sustainable caregiving dynamic.

Strategies to Strengthen Support Systems:

1. Regular Communication:
   - Strategy:
   - Regular and open communication fosters a sense of connection within the support system.
   - Patients and caregivers should discuss concerns, share updates, and express their feelings to maintain a strong bond.

2. Inclusion of Healthcare Providers:
   - Strategy:
   - Involving healthcare providers in the support system ensures a collaborative approach to managing the patient's health.
   - Regular check-ins with healthcare professionals contribute to a comprehensive understanding of the patient's needs.

3. Participation in Support Groups:
   - Strategy:
   - Both patients and caregivers benefit from participation in support groups.

- Sharing experiences, gaining insights, and learning from others strengthen the support system and provide a sense of community.

4. Educational Workshops and Resources:
   - Strategy:
   - Attend educational workshops or access resources provided by healthcare institutions.
   - Enhancing knowledge about pacemakers and related topics equips both patients and caregivers to navigate challenges more effectively.

5. Balancing Independence and Collaboration:
   - Strategy:
   - Striking a balance between maintaining independence and fostering collaboration is key.
   - Patients and caregivers should collaboratively make decisions, ensuring that the patient's autonomy is respected.

6. Prioritizing Self-Care for Caregivers:
   - Strategy:
   - Caregivers should prioritize their own self-care to prevent burnout.
   - Establishing boundaries, seeking support when needed, and taking breaks contribute to sustained caregiving.

7. Celebrating Milestones and Achievements:
   - Strategy:
   - Acknowledging and celebrating milestones, whether big or small, reinforces positive moments in the journey.

- Shared celebrations strengthen the bond between patients and caregivers.

Mental Health and Wellbeing

The profound impact of living with a pacemaker extends beyond the physical realm, influencing mental health and overall well-being.

Emotional Dimensions of Living with a Pacemaker:

1. Anxiety and Uncertainty:
   - Living with a pacemaker may evoke feelings of anxiety and uncertainty. The initial diagnosis, the implantation procedure, and concerns about the device's functioning can contribute to heightened levels of stress.

2. Adjustment and Acceptance:
   - Individuals may undergo a process of adjustment and acceptance, grappling with the reality of having a device implanted in their bodies. Accepting a change in one's health status can be emotionally challenging and may require time and support.

3. Identity and Self-Image:
   - The presence of a pacemaker may influence one's self-image and identity. Individuals may grapple with questions of normalcy, body image,

and how the device fits into their perception of themselves.

4. Fear of Complications:
  - Fear of complications, such as device malfunction or infections, can contribute to heightened stress levels. The potential impact of these complications on daily life and overall well-being may be a source of ongoing concern.

Coping Strategies for Mental Well-being:

1. Education and Understanding:
  - Understanding the pacemaker, its purpose, and the procedures involved can demystify the experience. Education empowers individuals to make informed decisions, alleviating anxiety stemming from uncertainty.

2. Open Communication:
  - Open communication with healthcare providers, loved ones, and support networks is crucial. Sharing concerns, fears, and feelings creates a supportive environment and fosters a sense of understanding.

3. Participation in Support Groups:
  - Joining support groups or connecting with individuals who have similar experiences can provide a sense of community. Shared experiences and mutual support contribute to emotional well-being.

4. Mindfulness and Stress Reduction Techniques:

-    Engaging in mindfulness practices, meditation, and stress reduction techniques can help manage anxiety. These practices promote a sense of calm and resilience in the face of life's challenges.

5. Professional Counseling:

- Seeking the guidance of mental health professionals or counselors offers a safe space to explore and address emotional concerns. Professional support can be instrumental in coping with anxiety, depression, or adjustment difficulties.

6. Embracing Positive Lifestyle Changes:

- Adopting positive lifestyle changes, including regular physical activity, a balanced diet, and adequate sleep, contributes to overall well-being. Physical health and mental health are interconnected, and a holistic approach supports both.

7. Empowerment through Self-Care:

- Prioritizing self-care is an empowering strategy. Engaging in activities that bring joy, setting realistic goals, and taking breaks when needed contribute to a positive mental outlook.

The Importance of Holistic Care:

1. Integrated Approach to Healthcare:

-    Holistic care recognizes the interconnectedness of physical and mental health.

Healthcare providers play a crucial role in adopting an integrated approach, addressing both the technical aspects of pacemaker care and the emotional well-being of patients.

2. Regular Mental Health Check-ins:

- Incorporating regular mental health check-ins into follow-up appointments ensures that emotional concerns are not overlooked. Healthcare providers can explore the emotional dimensions of living with a pacemaker and provide appropriate support.

3. Psychosocial Support Services:

- Access to psychosocial support services, including social workers or mental health professionals within healthcare institutions, enhances the support system for individuals with pacemakers.

4. Patient Education Programs:

- Patient education programs should extend beyond technical aspects to encompass the emotional dimensions of living with a pacemaker. Providing resources and information on mental health contributes to a more comprehensive understanding.

TRAVEL AND LIFESTYLE

"Not all those who wander are lost."
—J.R.R. Tolkien

Traveling with a Pacemaker

For individuals with pacemakers, the prospect of travel introduces considerations to ensure both safety and enjoyment.

Preparation and Planning:

1. Consultation with Healthcare Providers:

   - Pre-Travel Consultation: Before embarking on any journey, individuals with pacemakers should schedule a pre-travel consultation with their healthcare providers. This allows for a comprehensive assessment of the individual's health, the pacemaker's functioning, and any potential risks associated with travel.

2. Destination Research:

   - Understanding Local Healthcare Services: Researching the destination's healthcare infrastructure is crucial. Knowing the location of medical facilities, emergency services, and the availability of pacemaker clinics provides valuable information for any unforeseen circumstances.

3. Documentation and Identification:

- Carrying Medical Documentation: Individuals should carry essential medical documentation, including a pacemaker identification card, a letter from the healthcare provider detailing the device's specifications, and a list of current medications. These documents aid in seamless communication with security personnel and healthcare providers if needed.

Airport Security and Pacemaker Devices:

1. Communication with Security Personnel:

- Open Communication: Informing airport security personnel about the presence of a pacemaker is essential. Pacemaker devices may trigger metal detectors, and individuals should be prepared for additional screening procedures.

2. Handheld Metal Detectors and Body Scanners:

- Alternative Screening Options: While pacemakers are generally designed to withstand the electromagnetic fields of metal detectors and body scanners, individuals can request alternative screening methods, such as a pat-down or a handheld metal detector, to avoid prolonged exposure.

3. Carry Pacemaker Identification Card:

- Presentation of Identification Card: Presenting the pacemaker identification card and accompanying documentation facilitates a smoother screening process. Security personnel are trained to handle these situations, and clear communication is key to a stress-free experience.

In-Flight Considerations:

1. In-Flight Precautions:
   - Pacemaker Functioning and Altitude Changes: The functioning of a pacemaker is generally not affected by air travel. However, individuals should inform airline staff about the presence of a pacemaker. It's advisable to avoid placing electronic devices directly over the implant site and to use the opposite arm for carrying luggage or bags.

2. Carrying Medications and Essentials:
   - Hand-Carry Medications: Essential medications, including those related to the pacemaker, should be hand-carried in carry-on luggage. This ensures accessibility throughout the journey and minimizes the risk of loss or damage.

3. Hydration and Mobility:
   - Staying Hydrated: Maintaining hydration is crucial during air travel. Individuals should also engage in mild in-flight exercises, such as ankle circles and leg stretches, to promote circulation.

Accommodations and Local Support:

1. Choosing Accommodations:
   - Accessibility and Comfort: When selecting accommodations, consider factors such as

accessibility, proximity to medical facilities, and the availability of amenities that contribute to a comfortable stay.

2. Emergency Preparedness:

- Local Emergency Numbers: Familiarize yourself with local emergency numbers and the location of the nearest medical facilities. Having this information on hand enhances preparedness and swift response in case of emergencies.

3. Pacemaker Clinic Contacts:

- Identifying Pacemaker Clinics: Know the location and contact details of pacemaker clinics at the destination. In the rare event of device-related concerns, having access to specialized care ensures prompt attention.

Post-Travel Health Check:

1. Follow-Up Appointment:

- Post-Travel Health Check: Schedule a follow-up appointment with healthcare providers after returning from travel. This allows for a thorough assessment of the pacemaker's functioning and ensures any travel-related concerns are addressed.

Special Considerations
for Various Activities

While certain activities may require careful consideration and precautions, individuals with pacemakers can engage in a wide range of pursuits. This chapter explores special considerations for various activities, emphasizing the importance of informed decision-making, open communication with healthcare providers, and a proactive approach to well-being.

Physical Activities:

1. Moderate Exercise:
   - Individuals with pacemakers are generally encouraged to engage in moderate exercise. Activities like brisk walking, swimming, or cycling can contribute to cardiovascular health without putting undue stress on the device.

2. Avoiding Impact Sports:
   - High-impact sports, such as boxing or football, may pose a risk to the pacemaker and the leads. Individuals are advised to avoid such activities to prevent dislodgment or damage to the device.

3. Strength Training with Caution:
   - Strength training can be pursued with caution, focusing on lower weights and higher repetitions. Individuals should avoid placing heavy weights directly over the implant site.

4. Regular Monitoring:
   - Regular monitoring of heart rate during exercise is essential. Individuals can use heart rate monitors to ensure that their activity levels align with healthcare provider recommendations.

Recreational Activities:

1. Swimming and Water Activities:
   - Swimming is generally considered safe for individuals with pacemakers. However, caution is advised when engaging in water activities where the pacemaker may be submerged. Waterproof covers may be used for added protection.

2. Golfing and Non-Impact Sports:
   - Golfing, bowling, and other non-impact recreational activities are typically safe for individuals with pacemakers. It's essential to enjoy these pursuits while being mindful of any discomfort or unusual sensations.

3. Hiking and Outdoor Adventures:
   - Hiking and outdoor adventures are possible with a pacemaker. Individuals should be aware of their physical capabilities, choose trails that align with their fitness levels, and carry necessary medications and documentation.

Travel and Exploration:

1. Air Travel Precautions:
   - When traveling by air, individuals should inform airport security about the presence of a pacemaker. Carrying essential medical documentation, such as a pacemaker identification card, aids in streamlined security checks.

2. Access to Medical Facilities:
   - When planning travel, individuals should

consider the accessibility of medical facilities at their destination. Identifying pacemaker clinics and emergency services in advance contributes to preparedness.

3. Comfortable Accommodations:

- Selecting accommodations that prioritize comfort and accessibility enhances the overall travel experience. This includes proximity to medical facilities and the availability of amenities that cater to individual needs.

Work and Daily Activities:

1. Office and Desk Jobs:

- Individuals with pacemakers can typically continue with office jobs without major adjustments. However, prolonged periods of sitting should be interspersed with short breaks for movement.

2. Avoiding Heavy Lifting:

- Jobs that involve heavy lifting or strenuous physical activity may require modification. Individuals should communicate with employers to create a work environment that aligns with their health needs.

3. Routine Check-ups:

- Regular check-ups with healthcare providers are essential for monitoring the pacemaker's performance. Individuals should prioritize these appointments and communicate any changes in health or well-being promptly.

Social and Leisure Activities:

1. Dining Out and Socializing:
   - Dining out and socializing are generally unrestricted for individuals with pacemakers. However, being mindful of dietary choices, especially in terms of salt intake, contributes to overall heart health.

2. Participation in Community Events:
   - Engaging in community events, gatherings, and social activities is encouraged. Individuals should be aware of their energy levels, taking breaks as needed, and communicating openly with others about their health condition.

3. Mental Health and Leisure Pursuits:
   - Pursuits that contribute to mental well-being, such as attending cultural events, reading, or engaging in hobbies, are important. These activities enhance overall quality of life and should be pursued with enthusiasm.

INTERACTIONS WITH OTHER MEDICAL DEVICES

"The real question is not whether machines think but whether men do. The mystery which surrounds a thinking machine already surrounds a thinking man."
— B.F. Skinner

Precautions and Compatibility

The intricate nature of pacemakers necessitates careful consideration of their compatibility with other medical devices. Here we will discuss the precautions individuals with pacemakers should take concerning various medical devices, highlighting the importance of awareness, communication with healthcare providers, and maintaining harmony in health.

Understanding the Pacemaker:

1. Basic Functionality:
 - A pacemaker is a small, implanted device that regulates the heart's rhythm by delivering electrical impulses to the heart muscles. It consists of a generator, which contains the battery and

electronic circuits, and leads, which are thin wires connecting the generator to the heart.

2. Pacemaker Identification Card:

- Individuals with pacemakers are typically provided with a pacemaker identification card, detailing important information about the device, such as its make, model, and implantation date. This card is a valuable resource in emergency situations and for medical professionals.

Precautions and Compatibility:

1. Electronic Devices and Magnetic Fields:

- Precautions with Electronic Devices: Certain electronic devices can potentially interfere with pacemaker function. Individuals should maintain a safe distance from devices with strong magnets, such as MRI machines, as well as electronic gadgets like cell phones, which should be used on the side opposite the pacemaker.

2. Medical Procedures and Equipment:

- Precautions with Medical Procedures: Before undergoing any medical procedures, individuals should inform healthcare providers about the presence of a pacemaker. Certain procedures, such as magnetic resonance imaging (MRI) and electrocautery, may require specific precautions to prevent interference with the device.

3. Airport Security Screening:

- Communication at Airport Security: When

passing through airport security, individuals should inform security personnel about the pacemaker. While metal detectors are generally safe, individuals may undergo additional screening. Carrying the pacemaker identification card facilitates this process.

4. Mobile Phones and Electronic Gadgets:

- Maintaining Safe Distances: While the risk of interference with mobile phones is minimal, maintaining a safe distance (at least six inches) from the phone to the pacemaker site is recommended. Avoiding prolonged exposure and using the opposite ear for phone calls are additional precautions.

5. Household Appliances and Tools:

- Precautions in the Home: Common household appliances and tools, such as microwave ovens and power tools, are generally safe for individuals with pacemakers. However, maintaining caution and adhering to recommended distances ensure safety.

Communication with Healthcare Providers:

1. Regular Follow-up Appointments:

- Importance of Follow-up: Regular follow-up appointments with healthcare providers are crucial for monitoring the pacemaker's performance and ensuring compatibility with other medical devices. Adjustments to pacing parameters and updates on device technology may be addressed during these visits.

2. In-Depth Discussions:
   - Discussing Lifestyle and Activities: Individuals should engage in in-depth discussions with healthcare providers about their lifestyle, activities, and potential exposure to electronic devices. This information guides healthcare providers in providing personalized advice and ensuring optimal pacemaker function.

Advancements in Pacemaker Technology:

1. Shielding and Compatibility Features:
   - Technological Advancements: Modern pacemakers often incorporate advanced features, such as electromagnetic shielding, to enhance compatibility with various electronic devices. These technologies minimize the risk of interference, allowing individuals to confidently engage in daily activities.

2. Remote Monitoring Systems:
   - Remote Monitoring: Remote monitoring technology allows healthcare providers to monitor the pacemaker's performance remotely. This proactive approach enables early detection of issues, enhancing the overall safety and compatibility of the device with other medical technologies.

Communicating with

Healthcare Providers

Communication between individuals with pacemakers and their healthcare providers is the cornerstone of effective cardiac care. In the context of pacemakers, which are implanted devices designed to regulate heart rhythm, maintaining a robust line of communication is essential for optimal device function, ongoing monitoring, and addressing individual concerns.

Building a Foundation of Trust:

1. Understanding the Patient's Perspective:
   - Successful communication begins with healthcare providers understanding the unique perspective and experiences of individuals with pacemakers. Recognizing the emotional and practical aspects of living with a cardiac device fosters a supportive relationship.

2. Creating an Open and Non-judgmental Environment:
   - Establishing an environment that encourages open communication is paramount. Individuals should feel comfortable sharing their experiences, concerns, and questions without fear of judgment. A non-judgmental approach builds trust and strengthens the patient-provider partnership.

Importance of Regular Follow-up Appointments:

1. Monitoring Pacemaker Function:

-   Regular follow-up appointments allow healthcare providers to monitor the functioning of the pacemaker. These appointments include assessments of pacing parameters, battery life, and detection of any irregularities, ensuring the device is operating optimally.

2. Addressing Emerging Concerns:

- Follow-up appointments provide a platform for individuals to voice any emerging concerns or changes in their health. Open communication during these visits allows healthcare providers to address issues promptly, preventing potential complications.

3. Updating Health Information:

- Health conditions can evolve over time. Regular communication ensures that healthcare providers are updated on any changes in the individual's health, medications, or lifestyle, allowing for personalized and effective care.

Navigating Lifestyle and Activities:

1. Discussing Physical Activities:

- Individuals with pacemakers often engage in various physical activities. Clear communication about the types and intensities of exercise or activities is crucial for healthcare providers to offer tailored advice and ensure the safety of these pursuits.

2. Travel Plans and Precautions:

- Informing healthcare providers about upcoming travel plans is essential. Providers can offer guidance on potential challenges, recommend precautions, and ensure that individuals are adequately prepared for any medical needs while away from home.

Addressing Emotional Well-being:

1. Discussing Emotional Impact:

- Living with a pacemaker can have emotional implications. Discussing the emotional impact of the device, potential concerns, and coping strategies is crucial for comprehensive care. Healthcare providers can offer support and resources to address these aspects.

2. Mental Health Check-ins:

- Routine mental health check-ins should be incorporated into follow-up appointments. Addressing stress, anxiety, or any emotional challenges is an integral part of holistic care, contributing to overall well-being.

Empowering Individuals through Education:

1. Explaining Pacemaker Functionality:

- Educating individuals about the basic functionality of their pacemakers fosters empowerment. Understanding how the device works, its purpose, and potential considerations enables individuals to actively participate in their care.

2. Discussing Potential Interactions:

- Communication includes discussing potential interactions between the pacemaker and other aspects of life, such as electronic devices, medical procedures, and lifestyle choices. Educating individuals on precautions and best practices ensures safe and informed decision-making.

Embracing Shared Decision-Making:

1. Collaborative Decision-Making:

- Effective communication encourages collaborative decision-making. Individuals and healthcare providers working together to make decisions about treatment plans, lifestyle adjustments, and potential interventions promote a sense of shared responsibility.

2. Respecting Individual Preferences:

- Understanding and respecting the individual preferences of those with pacemakers is vital. Open dialogue allows healthcare providers to tailor care plans to align with the unique needs, values, and goals of each individual.

Utilizing Remote Monitoring Technology:

1. Advantages of Remote Monitoring:

- Remote monitoring technology enhances communication by allowing healthcare providers to remotely assess the performance of the pacemaker. This real-time data facilitates proactive intervention and reduces the need for frequent in-person appointments.

2. Regular Data Review:

- Regular review of remote monitoring data during follow-up appointments provides a comprehensive picture of the pacemaker's function. This enhances communication by allowing providers to address any issues promptly.

FINANCIAL AND INSURANCE CONSIDERATIONS

"If you want to know what God thinks of money, just look at the people he gave it to."
— Dorothy Parker

Cost of Pacemaker Implantation

It is essential to understand the financial aspects associated with this procedure. Let's discuss some important factors influencing the cost of pacemaker implantation, the components that contribute to the overall expenses, and considerations for individuals navigating the financial landscape of cardiac care.

Components of Pacemaker Implantation Costs:

1. Device Cost:
   - A significant portion of the overall cost is attributed to the pacemaker device itself. Pacemakers come in various models, each with unique features, and the cost varies accordingly. Newer models may incorporate advanced technologies, influencing the overall expense.

2. Surgical Procedure and Hospital Fees:

- The surgical procedure to implant the pacemaker is conducted in a hospital setting. Costs include surgical fees, charges for operating room use, anesthesia, and other associated hospital fees. The complexity of the procedure and the duration of the hospital stay contribute to these expenses.

3. Medical Professionals' Fees:

- The services of medical professionals involved in the pacemaker implantation, including the surgeon, anesthesiologist, and cardiologist, are billed separately. Their fees are integral components of the overall cost, reflecting their expertise and contributions to the procedure.

4. Diagnostic Tests and Pre-Operative Assessments:

- Pre-operative assessments, such as diagnostic tests and imaging studies, are conducted to evaluate the individual's overall health and suitability for the procedure. These tests contribute to the overall cost of pacemaker implantation.

5. Follow-up Care and Monitoring:

- Post-implantation care, including follow-up appointments, monitoring, and potential adjustments to the pacemaker settings, is an ongoing aspect of cardiac care. These follow-up services contribute to the overall cost and ensure the long-term functionality of the pacemaker.

Factors Influencing Cost Variations:

1. Geographic Location:
   - The cost of healthcare services can vary significantly based on the geographic location. Urban centers or regions with a higher cost of living may have higher healthcare expenses, impacting the overall cost of pacemaker implantation.

2. Hospital Facilities and Reputation:
   - The choice of hospital and its reputation for providing cardiac care services influence the cost. Hospitals with state-of-the-art facilities, renowned cardiac departments, and a track record of successful outcomes may have higher associated costs.

3. Type of Pacemaker:
   - The type and model of the pacemaker selected for implantation influence the overall cost. Advanced features, compatibility with remote monitoring technologies, and other functionalities contribute to variations in device costs.

4. Insurance Coverage:
   - The extent of insurance coverage plays a significant role in determining out-of-pocket expenses for individuals. Insurance plans may cover varying percentages of the total cost, impacting the financial responsibility of the patient.

5. Complications and Additional Interventions:

- The occurrence of complications during or after the implantation procedure may necessitate additional interventions, tests, or extended hospital stays. These unforeseen circumstances can contribute to increased costs.

Financial Considerations for Individuals:

1. Insurance Coverage Review:

- Individuals planning to undergo pacemaker implantation should carefully review their insurance coverage. Understanding the extent of coverage, including device costs, hospital fees, and professional services, is crucial for financial planning.

2. Pre-Authorization and Approval:

- Before the procedure, individuals should work closely with their healthcare providers to obtain pre-authorization and approval from their insurance providers. This ensures that the planned implantation is covered, reducing the risk of unexpected expenses.

3. Discussion with Healthcare Providers:

- Open communication with healthcare providers about financial concerns is essential. Individuals can discuss potential cost-saving measures, inquire about the availability of generic pacemaker models, and explore options for financial assistance or payment plans.

4. Utilizing Financial Assistance Programs:
   - Some hospitals and healthcare institutions offer financial assistance programs for individuals facing economic challenges. Exploring these options can provide relief for those with limited financial resources.

5. Comparing Costs and Seeking Second Opinions:
   - Individuals can explore cost variations by obtaining estimates from multiple healthcare providers or hospitals. Seeking second opinions can provide a comprehensive understanding of potential treatment options and associated costs.

Insurance Coverage and Reimbursement

As with any medical procedure, understanding the landscape of insurance coverage and reimbursement is paramount. This essay explores the intricacies of insurance coverage for pacemaker implantation, factors influencing reimbursement, and the importance of navigating the financial aspects of cardiac care to ensure optimal outcomes for both patients and healthcare providers.

Overview of Pacemaker Implantation:

1. Role of Pacemakers:
   - Pacemakers are electronic devices implanted

in the chest to regulate the heart's rhythm by delivering electrical impulses. They play a crucial role in managing arrhythmias and enhancing the overall quality of life for individuals with specific cardiac conditions.

2. Medical Necessity and Decision-making:

- The decision to implant a pacemaker is guided by medical necessity. Healthcare providers assess the individual's health status, the severity of the cardiac condition, and the potential benefits of the device. This medical evaluation is fundamental to justifying the need for the procedure.

Insurance Coverage for Pacemaker Implantation:

1. Types of Insurance Plans:

- Insurance coverage for pacemaker implantation varies based on the type of insurance plan individuals have. Common types include private health insurance, government-sponsored plans (such as Medicare and Medicaid), and employer-sponsored health insurance.

2. Coverage Components:

- Insurance coverage for pacemaker implantation typically includes various components:

- Device Cost: Coverage for the pacemaker device itself, which constitutes a significant portion of the overall cost.

- Hospital Fees: Coverage for the surgical procedure, operating room use, anesthesia, and associated hospital fees.

- Professional Fees: Coverage for the services of medical professionals, including the surgeon, anesthesiologist, and cardiologist.

3. Pre-authorization and Approval:

- Before undergoing the procedure, individuals are advised to work closely with their healthcare providers to obtain pre-authorization and approval from their insurance providers. This involves submitting documentation that justifies the medical necessity of the pacemaker implantation.

4. In-Network vs. Out-of-Network Providers:

- The choice of healthcare providers can impact coverage. In-network providers are generally preferred, as they have negotiated rates with insurance companies. Out-of-network providers may result in higher out-of-pocket expenses for individuals.

5. Coverage Limitations and Exclusions:

- Insurance plans may have limitations or exclusions related to pacemaker implantation. Individuals should carefully review their policy documents to understand any specific conditions or circumstances that may affect coverage.

Reimbursement Process:

1. Submission of Claims:

- Following the pacemaker implantation,

healthcare providers submit claims to the insurance company for reimbursement. These claims include detailed information about the procedure, associated costs, and documentation supporting the medical necessity of the intervention.

2. Adjudication and Payment:

- The insurance company reviews the submitted claims through a process called adjudication. During adjudication, the company assesses whether the services provided align with the terms of the insurance policy. Once approved, reimbursement is processed, and payment is made to the healthcare providers.

3. Patient Responsibility:

- Despite insurance coverage, individuals may still have out-of-pocket expenses. Patient responsibility includes deductibles, co-payments, and co-insurance, which vary based on the specific insurance plan. Understanding these financial responsibilities is crucial for financial planning.

4. Appeals Process:

- In cases where claims are denied or disputed, individuals have the right to appeal the decision. The appeals process allows for a reevaluation of the claim, providing an opportunity to present additional information or address any discrepancies.

Factors Influencing Reimbursement:

1. Medical Necessity and Documentation:

- Clear documentation supporting the medical necessity of pacemaker implantation is fundamental for reimbursement. Healthcare providers must provide detailed records outlining the individual's health status, diagnostic tests, and the rationale for the procedure.

2. Coding Accuracy:

- Accurate coding of the procedure and associated services is crucial for reimbursement. Medical billing codes specify the interventions performed and help insurance companies categorize and process claims efficiently.

3. In-Network vs. Out-of-Network Reimbursement:

- Reimbursement rates for in-network and out-of-network providers may differ. In-network providers generally have established agreements with insurance companies, leading to negotiated reimbursement rates. Out-of-network providers may receive lower reimbursement.

4. Timely Submission of Claims:

- Timely submission of claims is essential for efficient reimbursement. Delays in claim submission may result in complications, and adherence to insurance company deadlines is critical for a smooth reimbursement process.

Patient Advocacy and Financial Planning:

1. Understanding Insurance Policies:

- Individuals are encouraged to thoroughly understand the terms and conditions of their insurance policies. This includes coverage limitations, exclusions, and any potential financial responsibilities.

2. Communication with Healthcare Providers:

- Open communication with healthcare providers about insurance coverage is crucial. Providers can assist individuals in navigating the reimbursement process, providing necessary documentation, and addressing any concerns.

3. Financial Counseling Services:

- Some healthcare institutions offer financial counseling services to assist individuals in understanding and managing the financial aspects of medical procedures. These services can provide valuable guidance on payment plans, financial assistance programs, and available resources.

4. Advance Planning for Out-of-Pocket Costs:

- Individuals should plan for potential out-of-pocket costs associated with pacemaker implantation. This includes setting aside funds for deductibles, co-payments, and any other financial responsibilities specified in their insurance plan.

COMMUNITY AND
SUPPORT GROUPS

"It seems to me that trying to live without friends is like milking a bear to get cream for your morning coffee. It is a whole lot of trouble, and then not worth much after get it."
-Zora Neal Hurston

Joining Support Networks

The journey of living with a pacemaker is not one that individuals need to embark on alone. Joining support networks can provide an invaluable source of encouragement, information, and shared experiences.

Emotional Support:

1. Shared Experiences and Empathy:
-   Joining a support network connects individuals with others who have undergone pacemaker implantation. Sharing experiences and hearing stories from those who have walked a similar path fosters empathy, understanding, and a sense of community.

2. Coping with Emotional Challenges:
-   The emotional impact of living with a

pacemaker, whether it's adjusting to a new reality or managing anxiety, can be challenging. Support networks provide a safe space for individuals to express their feelings, receive validation, and gain insights into coping strategies.

3. Reducing Feelings of Isolation:

- Living with a cardiac device can sometimes lead to feelings of isolation. Support networks create a sense of belonging, helping individuals realize they are not alone in their journey. This shared camaraderie promotes emotional well-being.

Educational Resources:

1. Information Sharing:

- Support networks serve as valuable platforms for sharing information. Individuals can exchange knowledge about pacemakers, cardiac health, and lifestyle adjustments. This collective wisdom enhances the overall understanding of living with a pacemaker.

2. Access to Expertise:

- Support networks often include individuals with diverse backgrounds, including healthcare professionals, who can provide insights and answer questions. This access to expertise empowers individuals with reliable information and helps them make informed decisions.

3. Learning from Others' Experiences:

- Hearing about the experiences of others who have undergone pacemaker implantation provides practical insights into what to expect before, during, and after the procedure. This firsthand knowledge is often more relatable and valuable than medical literature.

Practical Advice and Tips:

1. Daily Living Strategies:
- Support networks offer practical advice on navigating daily life with a pacemaker. From tips on managing electronic devices to insights into maintaining an active lifestyle, individuals can benefit from the collective wisdom of the group.

2. Dealing with Challenges:
- Challenges, such as adjusting to lifestyle changes, travel considerations, or handling medical appointments, are part of the journey with a pacemaker. Support networks provide a forum for discussing these challenges and brainstorming effective solutions.

3. Real-life Perspectives:
- While medical professionals provide essential guidance, real-life perspectives from individuals who have experienced similar challenges offer a unique and relatable dimension. Support networks bridge the gap between medical advice and practical, day-to-day living.

Building a Supportive Community:

1. Peer-to-Peer Encouragement:

- Support networks create a platform for individuals to encourage each other. Whether it's celebrating milestones, offering words of encouragement during challenging times, or simply being there to listen, the peer-to-peer support is invaluable.

2. Community Events and Gatherings:

- Many support networks organize community events, gatherings, or online forums where members can meet in person or virtually. These events foster a sense of community, allowing individuals to strengthen their connections beyond digital interactions.

3. Advocacy and Awareness:

- Support networks often engage in advocacy efforts to raise awareness about cardiac health and the experiences of individuals living with pacemakers. By participating in these initiatives, individuals contribute to a broader understanding of cardiac conditions.

Overcoming Stigma and Fear:

1. Addressing Stigma:

- Support networks play a crucial role in addressing the stigma sometimes associated with cardiac devices. By openly discussing experiences, individuals can challenge misconceptions and create a more inclusive and understanding environment.

2. Empowering Through Shared Stories:
    - Shared stories within the support network can be empowering. Individuals who have overcome challenges and embraced life with a pacemaker inspire others to face their fears, fostering a positive and resilient mindset.

Sharing Experiences with Others

Living with a pacemaker is a unique journey that brings both challenges and triumphs. The act of sharing one's experiences with others, whether through personal conversations, support groups, or online platforms, holds immense significance.

Therapeutic Catharsis:

1. Emotional Release and Validation:
    - Sharing pacemaker experiences provides a therapeutic outlet for individuals to express their emotions. Narrating one's journey, challenges, and victories serves as a form of emotional release, allowing individuals to validate their feelings and experiences.

2. Coping with Uncertainty:
    - The act of sharing becomes a coping mechanism, particularly in dealing with the uncertainty that often accompanies living with

a pacemaker. Expressing fears, anxieties, and uncertainties fosters a sense of control and resilience.

3. Connecting with Others:

- Individuals who share their experiences often find that they connect with others on a deeper level. This shared connection forms a supportive network, breaking down the walls of isolation that can sometimes accompany cardiac conditions.

Educational Insights:

1. Real-life Perspectives:

- Narratives about living with a pacemaker offer real-life perspectives that go beyond medical textbooks. These insights into day-to-day experiences provide a nuanced understanding of the challenges and adjustments individuals face.

2. Practical Tips and Advice:

- Sharing experiences allows individuals to offer practical tips and advice to others who may be on a similar journey. From managing daily activities to coping with emotional aspects, these shared tips contribute to a collective pool of knowledge.

3. Awareness and Understanding:

- Personal narratives contribute to raising awareness and understanding about pacemakers and cardiac health. By sharing experiences, individuals become advocates, demystifying the condition and fostering a more informed and compassionate society.

Building Empathy and Support:

1. Fostering Empathy:
   - Listening to others' pacemaker experiences fosters empathy. Understanding the challenges and triumphs of fellow individuals cultivates a compassionate mindset, creating a supportive environment that extends beyond the immediate community.

2. Offering Encouragement:
   - Sharing personal stories of overcoming challenges with a pacemaker provides encouragement to those who may be navigating similar paths. Encouragement becomes a powerful tool for motivating individuals to face their own situations with resilience.

3. Breaking Down Stigmas:
   - The open sharing of pacemaker experiences contributes to breaking down stigmas associated with cardiac conditions. By humanizing the experience and presenting it as a shared reality, individuals challenge stereotypes and promote inclusivity.

Online Platforms and Support Groups:

1. Global Connections:
   - Online platforms and support groups create opportunities for individuals worldwide to share their pacemaker experiences. This global

connection allows for a diverse range of stories, fostering a sense of unity among individuals with different backgrounds and experiences.

2. 24/7 Support:

- Virtual communities provide a continuous source of support. Individuals can share their experiences, seek advice, and offer encouragement at any time, creating a dynamic and accessible network that aligns with the diverse needs of its members.

3. Anonymity and Openness:

- Online platforms often allow for a level of anonymity, encouraging individuals to share their experiences more openly. This freedom of expression can lead to more candid discussions, creating a safe space for vulnerability.

Promoting Positive Mental Health:

1. Reducing Isolation and Loneliness:

- One of the significant impacts of sharing pacemaker experiences is the reduction of isolation and loneliness. Knowing that others have faced similar challenges and triumphed creates a sense of solidarity, fostering positive mental health.

2. Celebrating Milestones:

- Celebrating personal milestones, whether big or small, becomes a collective joy within a supportive community. Sharing achievements and positive moments reinforces a sense of accomplishment and resilience.

3. Supportive Network for Mental Well-being:

- Being part of a community that shares pacemaker experiences creates a supportive network for mental well-being. Individuals can turn to this network during moments of emotional turbulence, finding understanding and encouragement.

FUTURE DEVELOPMENTS IN PACEMAKER TECHNOLOGY

"Life can only be understood backwards; but it must be lived forwards."
— Søren Kierkegaard

Emerging Trends and Innovations

Pacemaker technology has undergone remarkable advancements over the years, transforming the landscape of cardiac care and enhancing the quality of life for individuals with heart rhythm disorders.

Miniaturization and Leadless Pacemakers:

1. Introduction to Leadless Technology:
   - A groundbreaking innovation in pacemaker technology is the development of leadless pacemakers. Unlike traditional pacemakers that require leads (wires) threaded through veins to the heart, leadless pacemakers are self-contained devices placed directly in the heart's chambers.

2. Advantages of Leadless Pacemakers:
   - Leadless pacemakers offer several advantages,

including a reduced risk of lead-related complications, simpler implantation procedures, and a more aesthetically pleasing solution for patients. This innovation represents a significant leap forward in improving the safety and efficiency of cardiac pacing.

Wireless Communication and Remote Monitoring:

1. Advancements in Remote Monitoring:

- Modern pacemakers are equipped with wireless communication capabilities, allowing for remote monitoring of the device's functionality. This technology enables healthcare providers to access real-time data, enhancing the management of patients' cardiac health.

2. Benefits of Remote Monitoring:

- Remote monitoring offers several benefits, including early detection of potential issues, timely intervention, and reduced need for in-person clinic visits. Patients can enjoy the convenience of being monitored from the comfort of their homes, improving overall healthcare accessibility.

Closed-Loop Stimulation:

1. Enhanced Physiological Pacing:

- Closed-loop stimulation is an innovative pacing technology that adjusts the heart rate in response to physiological cues, such as changes in physical activity or stress. This adaptive approach provides a more natural and responsive pacing solution, closely mimicking the body's intrinsic regulatory mechanisms.

2. Optimizing Energy Efficiency:

- Closed-loop stimulation not only enhances physiological pacing but also optimizes energy efficiency. By tailoring pacing rates to the body's demands, this technology conserves battery life, reducing the frequency of device replacements and associated surgeries.

Magnetic Resonance Imaging (MRI) Compatibility:

1. Overcoming Historical Limitations:

- Traditionally, pacemaker recipients faced limitations when it came to undergoing magnetic resonance imaging (MRI) scans. However, recent innovations have led to the development of MRI-compatible pacemakers, allowing individuals to benefit from essential diagnostic imaging without compromising device function.

2. Expanding Diagnostic Possibilities:

- MRI-compatible pacemakers expand diagnostic possibilities for individuals with pacemakers, providing healthcare providers with clearer insights into various medical conditions. This breakthrough underscores the commitment to improving overall patient care and diagnostic capabilities.

Energy Harvesting and Battery Longevity:

1. Harvesting Body Energy:

- Energy harvesting is an emerging trend that explores the possibility of generating power for pacemakers from the body's natural movements. This innovation aims to reduce or eliminate the need for battery replacements by harnessing energy from the environment within the body.

2. Extending Battery Life:

- Prolonging battery life is a critical aspect of pacemaker technology. Innovations in battery technology, coupled with energy harvesting, have the potential to significantly extend the lifespan of pacemaker batteries, reducing the frequency of surgical interventions.

Artificial Intelligence (AI) Integration:

1. Smart Pacing Algorithms:

- The integration of artificial intelligence into pacemaker technology introduces smart pacing algorithms. These algorithms analyze data from the pacemaker and make real-time adjustments to pacing parameters based on the individual's physiological needs, contributing to personalized and adaptive pacing strategies.

2. Predictive Analytics for Health Monitoring:

- AI-powered pacemakers can employ predictive analytics to anticipate potential health issues, allowing for proactive intervention. This capability enhances the device's role not only in cardiac pacing but also in comprehensive health monitoring and preventive care.

Potential Advancements in Pacemaker Technology

Now we will explore the potential advancements in pacemaker technology that hold the promise of reshaping the landscape of cardiac pacing, ushering in an era of improved functionality, patient-centered care, and enhanced longevity of devices.

Next-Generation Materials and Biocompatibility:

1. Innovative Material Science:
  - The integration of advanced materials into pacemaker design is a potential avenue for improvement. Next-generation materials with superior strength, flexibility, and biocompatibility may pave the way for pacemakers that are more resilient, adaptable to physiological changes, and comfortable for patients.

2. Bioengineered Coatings:
  - Bioengineered coatings can enhance the compatibility of pacemaker components with the body, reducing the risk of adverse reactions and promoting tissue integration. This could lead to pacemakers that are not only functional but also seamlessly integrate into the natural cardiac environment.

Gene Therapy and Biological Pacing:

1. Revolutionizing Cardiac Pacing:
   - Gene therapy holds immense potential for revolutionizing cardiac pacing. By targeting specific genes related to electrical signaling in the heart, researchers aim to develop biological pacing techniques that could eliminate the need for electronic devices. This groundbreaking approach could provide a natural and dynamic solution for regulating heart rhythm.

2. Tailored Genetic Interventions:
   - Personalized gene therapies may become a reality, allowing healthcare providers to tailor interventions based on an individual's genetic makeup. This level of precision could address the unique needs of each patient, leading to more effective and patient-specific cardiac pacing solutions.

Regenerative Medicine and Tissue Engineering:

1. Regenerating Cardiac Tissue:
   - Advancements in regenerative medicine and tissue engineering may offer the possibility of regenerating damaged cardiac tissue. This could have profound implications for individuals with heart conditions, potentially reducing the need for electronic pacing devices by promoting natural healing and regeneration.

2. Biological Pacemaker Cells:

- Research in tissue engineering is exploring the development of biological pacemaker cells that can mimic the natural pacemaking function of the heart. These cells, when integrated into the cardiac tissue, could serve as biological pacemakers, offering a novel and regenerative approach to cardiac pacing.

Advanced Sensing and Signal Processing:

1. Multimodal Sensing Capabilities:

- Future pacemakers may incorporate advanced sensing technologies that go beyond traditional methods. Multimodal sensing capabilities could enable pacemakers to gather a more comprehensive range of physiological data, allowing for a nuanced understanding of the patient's overall health.

2. Signal Processing Algorithms:

- Enhanced signal processing algorithms could refine the interpretation of cardiac signals, enabling pacemakers to respond more precisely to the body's needs. This could result in adaptive pacing strategies that optimize energy efficiency and improve the overall performance of the device.

Artificial Intelligence and Machine Learning Integration:

1. Predictive Analytics for Health Monitoring:

- The integration of artificial intelligence

and machine learning holds the potential for predictive analytics in health monitoring. Pacemakers equipped with intelligent algorithms could anticipate changes in the patient's condition, allowing for proactive intervention and preventive care.

2. Learning-Based Adaptation:

- Machine learning algorithms could enable pacemakers to learn and adapt to the individual patient's lifestyle and physiological patterns over time. This adaptive capability would contribute to a more personalized and responsive pacing strategy, aligning with the dynamic nature of each patient's health.

Energy Harvesting and Sustainable Power Sources:

1. Advancements in Energy Harvesting:

- Continued advancements in energy harvesting technologies may address the perennial challenge of pacemaker battery life. Innovations in harvesting ambient energy from the body or external sources could significantly extend the longevity of pacemaker batteries, reducing the need for frequent replacements.

2. Implantable Power Sources:

- Exploration of novel implantable power sources, such as biofuel cells or miniature generators, may offer sustainable alternatives to traditional batteries. These innovative power solutions could contribute to the development of eco-friendly and long-lasting pacemaker devices.

Neuromodulation and Autonomic Regulation:

1. Neural Interface Technologies:
-    The   integration   of   neuromodulation technologies may enable pacemakers to interact with the autonomic nervous system. This could lead to advanced pacing strategies that dynamically regulate heart rate based on real-time neural signals, providing a more holistic approach to cardiac care.

2. Closed-Loop Systems:
- Closed-loop systems that interface with neural signals could create feedback loops, allowing pacemakers to modulate pacing parameters in response to changes in the body's autonomic state. This level of sophistication could contribute to improved physiological pacing and overall patient well-being.

GLOSSARY

"No book can ever be finished. While working on it we learn just enough to find it immature the moment we turn away from it"
— *Karl Popper*

1. Pacemaker: A small, implantable medical device that regulates and controls the heart's rhythm by delivering electrical impulses to the heart muscles.

2. Pulse Generator: The core component of a pacemaker, housing the electronic circuitry, programmable settings, and the power source (battery) necessary for generating electrical impulses.

3. Leads: Insulated wires that connect the pulse generator to specific chambers of the heart, facilitating the transmission of electrical impulses and enabling the pacemaker to regulate heart rhythm.

4. Atrium: One of the two upper chambers of the heart responsible for receiving blood from the veins and pumping it into the ventricles.

5. Ventricles: The two lower chambers of the heart that pump blood to the lungs (right ventricle) and

the rest of the body (left ventricle).

6. Arrhythmias: Irregular heart rhythms that can result in the heart beating too fast (tachycardia) or too slow (bradycardia), often necessitating pacemaker intervention.

7. Heart Failure: A condition where the heart is unable to pump blood effectively, potentially leading to arrhythmias and requiring pacemaker support.

8. Bradycardia: A condition characterized by an abnormally slow heart rate, often requiring pacemaker intervention to restore a normal rhythm.

9. Heart Block: A condition where the electrical signals that regulate heart rhythm are delayed or blocked, often necessitating pacemaker implantation.

10. Closed-Loop Stimulation: An innovative pacing technology that adjusts heart rate based on physiological cues, providing a more natural and adaptive pacing strategy.

11. Magnetic Resonance Imaging (MRI) Compatibility: The ability of a pacemaker to withstand and function properly during an MRI scan, a crucial consideration in modern pacemaker design.

12. Energy Harvesting: The process of capturing

and utilizing ambient energy, potentially harnessed within the body, to power pacemakers and extend battery life.

13. Artificial Intelligence (AI) Integration: The incorporation of AI algorithms into pacemaker technology, enabling real-time adjustments to pacing parameters based on the patient's physiological needs.

14. Leadless Pacemakers: Pacemakers that do not require leads and are implanted directly into the heart, reducing the risk of lead-related complications.

15. Gene Therapy: A therapeutic approach that involves manipulating the genes associated with cardiac pacing to develop biological pacing solutions.

16. Regenerative Medicine: A field exploring the use of stem cells and tissue engineering to repair or replace damaged cardiac tissue, potentially reducing the need for electronic pacing devices.

17. Multimodal Sensing: The incorporation of advanced sensing technologies in pacemakers to gather a more comprehensive range of physiological data for nuanced pacing adjustments.

18. Remote Monitoring Technology: The utilization of wireless communication to remotely monitor pacemaker function, enabling healthcare

providers to access real-time data and intervene when necessary.

19. Energy Harvesting: A technology that explores the possibility of generating power for pacemakers from the body's natural movements or external sources, reducing the need for battery replacements.

20. Closed-Loop Stimulation: An adaptive pacing technology that adjusts heart rate based on physiological cues, optimizing energy efficiency and providing a more natural pacing strategy.

21. Bioengineered Coatings: Specialized coatings on pacemaker components to enhance biocompatibility, reducing the risk of adverse reactions and promoting integration with surrounding tissues.

22. Implantable Power Sources: Innovative power sources, such as biofuel cells or energy-harvesting technologies, explored to extend the longevity of pacemakers and reduce the need for frequent battery replacements.

23. Telehealth: The use of telecommunications technology to provide healthcare services remotely, allowing patients with pacemakers to receive virtual consultations and monitoring.

24. Wearable Devices: External devices worn by patients that can monitor and transmit data related to pacemaker function and overall

health, enhancing continuous care and patient engagement.